OSCE and OSPE in
Physiology

A Competency Assessment Tool

According to the latest CBME Guidelines | Competency Based Undergraduate Curriculum for the Indian Medical Graduate

OSCE and OSPE in
Physiology

A Competency Assessment Tool

According to the latest CBME Guidelines | Competency Based Undergraduate Curriculum for the Indian Medical Graduate

Tripti Srivastava Waghmare
MBBS, MD, FAIMER, AFAMEE, MPhil, PhD

Professor, Department of Physiology
Director, Internal Quality Assurance Cell (IQAC)
DMIMS (DU)
Convener, MCI Nodal Centre for
National Faculty Development
Member, Fac Dev Committee, AMEE
Jawaharlal Nehru Medical College
Datta Meghe Institute of Medical Sciences
Sawangi (M), Wardha, Maharashtra, India
Email: drtriptisrivastava@gmail.com

Alka Rawekar
MBBS, MD, MPhil, FAIMER, PhD

Professor, Department of Physiology
Dean, School of Allied Health Sciences, DMIMS (DU)
Co-Convener, MCI Nodal Centre for National Faculty
Development
Jawaharlal Nehru Medical College
Datta Meghe Institute of Medical Sciences
Sawangi (M), Wardha, Maharashtra, India
Email: alka.rawekar@gmail.com

Arunita Jagzape
MBBS, MD, MPhil, FAIMER, PhD (Physiology)

Assistant Professor, Department of Physiology
All India Institute of Medical Sciences
Raipur, Chhattisgarh
Email: arunitaj4@gmail.com

Lalitbhushan Waghmare
MBBS, MD, MPhil, PhD

Professor, Department of Physiology
Pro-Vice-Chancellor
Datta Meghe Institute of Medical Sciences
Sawangi (M), Wardha, Maharashtra, India
Email: drlalitwaghmare@gmail.com

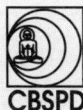

CBSPD

CBS Publishers & Distributors Pvt Ltd
New Delhi • Bengaluru • Chennai • Kochi • Kolkata • Lucknow • Mumbai
Hyderabad • Jharkhand • Nagpur • Patna • Pune • Uttarakhand

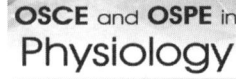

OSCE and **OSPE** in
Physiology
A Competency Assessment Tool

ISBN: 978-81-948986-5-8

Copyright © Authors and Publisher

First Edition: 2021

Reprint: 2024

Published by Satish Kumar Jain and produced by Varun Jain for

CBS Publishers & Distributors Pvt Ltd

4819/XI Prahlad Street, 24 Ansari Road, Daryaganj, New Delhi 110 002, India
Ph: 011-23289259, 23266861   Website: www.cbspd.com
                                                        e-mail: delhi@cbspd.com
Corporate Office: 204 FIE, Industrial Area, Patparganj, Delhi 110 092, India
Ph: 011-4934 4934   Fax: 011-4934 4935   e-mail: publishing@cbspd.com; publicity@cbspd.com

Branches

- **Bengaluru:** Seema House 2975, 17th Cross, K.R. Road, Banasankari 2nd Stage, Bengaluru 560 070, Karnataka, India
  Ph: +91-80-26771678/79   Fax: +91-80-26771680   e-mail: bangalore@cbspd.com
- **Chennai:** 7, Subbaraya Street, Shenoy Nagar, Chennai 600 030, Tamil Nadu, India
  Ph: +91-44-26680620, 26681266   Fax: +91-44-42032115   e-mail: chennai@cbspd.com
- **Kochi:** 42/1325, 1326, Power House Road, Opposite KSEB, Power House, Ernakulam 682018, Kochi, Kerala, India
  Ph: +91-484-4059061–65, 67   Fax: +91-484-4059065   e-mail: kochi@cbspd.com
- **Kolkata:** 147, Hind Ceramics Compound, 1st Floor, Nilgunj Road, Belghoria, Kolkata 700056, West Bengal, India
  Ph: +91-33-25633055/56   e-mail: kolkata@cbspd.com
- **Lucknow:** Basement, Khushnuma Complex, 7 Meerabai Marg (behind Jawahar Bhawan), Lucknow 226001, UP, India
  Ph: +91-522-4000032   e-mail: tiwari.lucknow@cbspd.com
- **Mumbai:** PWD Shed, Gala No. 25/26, Ramchandra Bhatt Marg, Next to JJ Hospital, Gate No. 2, Opp. Union Bank of India, Noorbaug
  Mumbai 400009, Maharashtra, India
  Ph: +91-22-66661880/89   e-mail: mumbai@cbspd.com

Representatives

- **Hyderabad**   0-9885175004
- **Patna**   0-9334159340
- **Jharkhand**   0-9811541605
- **Pune**   0-9664372571
- **Nagpur**   0-8692091830
- **Uttarakhand**   0-9716462459

Printed at: Mudrak, Noida, UP, India

Foreword

Health has always been perceived as the fundamental right attributable to every global citizen. The genuine actualization of this contemplated goal mandates effective and meaningful generation of trained health manpower in required numbers with efficacy and capacity.

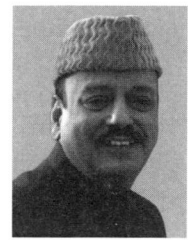

Healthcare delivery system and its efficiency is totally dependent on the efficacy of the trained health manpower generated by the various medical schools in any country. It is for this very reason it is imperative that standards of medical education must be so set out that they are capable of mitigating these vital challenges, concerns and need in the most desired manner in the larger interest of men, mankind and humanity as a whole.

It is on this advent that Competency Based Undergraduate Medical Education was envisioned and the same has been put into vogue in order to make medical education a bonafide instrumentality of actualizing the mandated 'Welfare State' embedded in the Constitution of India for the fulfillment of legitimate expectations of all its citizens.

One of the important aspects of this paradigm shift contemplated through Competency Based Medical Education Curriculum is structuring of the core competencies, their blending with ancillary ones and making them progress in the context of ascendancy thereto and their appropriate certification in an objective and credible manner. This mandates an integrated approach for the fulfillment of so set out objectives in their entirety.

It is in this backdrop the significance of the book titled *OSCE and OSPE in Physiology: A Competency Assessment Tool* authored by Dr. Tripti Srivastava, Professor of Physiology and Convener of the Nodal Centre recognized by the Medical Council of India; Dr. Alka Rawekar, Professor of Physiology and Co-Convener of the MCI Nodal Centre; Dr. Arunita Jagzape, Assistant Professor, Physiology at All India Institute of Medical Sciences, Raipur; and Dr. Lalit Waghmare, Professor, Physiology and Pro-Vice-Chancellor, DMIMS; turns out to be a pioneer work of its type aimed at fulfilling the acutely felt and perceived necessities.

The inclusions in the book have been diligently planned and appropriately structured. They have been evolved to give an operational shape to the modality of Objectively Structured Clinical Examination (OSCE) in order to give real meaning and essence to the hitherto operational phrase that the entire medicine and its allied specialities are based on the core edifice of physiology and biochemistry. The diligence with which this core edifice is strengthened is directly proportional to the efficacy of the suprastructure placed thereon.

The creative manifestation so diligently brought out by the authors is not only timely and relevant, but is also bound to act as a ready reckoner to all the concerned in order to make the teaching and learning of physiology purposive, meaningful, cogent, credible, consistent and relevant to the targeted purpose and ending up in being impactful.

This kaleidoscope of objectives to my understanding would get fulfilled and actualized by this notable creative creation by the authors in the form of this book, which has the peculiarity of appropriate syntaxing and having a free-flowing character proving to be of handy use to all the end users and thereby establishing its own sense of utility.

The authors deserve all compliments and appreciation for their notable initiative, which is the saga of the trinity of their unparalleled devotion, emulative dedication and unending commitment.

I am sure the testimony by the users would be a real pragmatic recognition to this glorious creativity. I record my humble gratitude to the authors for their laudable and notable effort, which to my perception is bound to fill in the huge void, which is in vogue, but would stands filled up by this notable initiative and manifestation thereto.

Vedprakash Mishra
Pro-Chancellor,
Datta Meghe Institute of Medical Sciences (DU)
Sawangi (M), Wardha, Maharashtra, India

Preface

Greetings to all our revered readers.

This book, *OSCE and OSPE in Physiology: A Competency Assessment Tool*, is a reflection of our ardent urge to provide a path to the concepts and execution of OSCE at the end user level. This book will cater to medical, dental students as beneficiaries and not just limited to them, it can extend to other health professionals dealing with the patients. The book shall help the students to prepare for the assessment of competencies and provide learning opportunity as well.

Dear venerated readers, this book is not a closed system but an open sea of dynamic explorations wherein you as a reader can ratify to run your imaginations and modifications and carry the concepts beyond this book instead of ending your quest of experimentation with a deadlock.

We have tried to include the details of OSCE procedural stations and response stations spanning respiratory system, cardiovascular system, abdomen and central nervous system. We have also included some of the OSPE procedural stations for hematology practicals, clinical photographs, and problem-solving questions.

The marks allotted to the items in checklist are as per our best knowledge and understanding (which can be modified as per your ideation). We have provided with the correction factor for every station. This can be explained with the following example:

Total marks allotted to all OSCE stations are 40 and hence for every station, it will be 4, if the number of stations are 10. Total number of stations are 12 that includes 5 procedural station, 5 response stations (total 10) and 2 rest stations and total marks allotted for procedural stations are 15, 16, 23, 10, 15 respectively and for response stations are 4 each.

But the marks allotted for each station are unique and different. Therefore, we calculate the correction factor for every station. If the marks allotted to one station is 15 and we have to reduce it to 4, then the correction factor will be $4/15 = 0.26$. For 16 marks station, it will be $4/16 = 0.25$; for 23, $4/23 = 0.17$ and so on.

We have included 5 scale format of Global Rating as well; "1. Poor; 2. Unsatisfactory; 3. Satisfactory; 4. Good; 5. Excellent". The Global Rating can also be executed using 3 scales.

In this way, we can customized the marks for every station for each student.

We wish all our readers a pleasant reading through this book and we welcome feedback from our readers regarding this book.

Tripti Srivastava Waghmare
Alka Rawekar
Arunita Jagzape
Lalitbhushan Waghmare

Contents

Introduction

"Education is not teaching students what they do not know but making them behave as they do not behave"

Ruskin

Need for OSCE

MCI aims at a competent Indian Medical Graduate since 2015, through competency-based education and the assessment of these acquired competencies. The traditional tools of assessment for practical skills had their own advantages and challenges that are as follows:

a. *Short case examinations*: In short case examinations of 15 to 20 minutes per patient, candidates are asked to perform a brief and focused history and clinical examination with specific clinical findings. The case is discussed over 5 to 10 minutes with the examiners in an unstructured manner of marking. Different candidates examine different patients thus affecting the standardization. Short case examination has an advantage of real patient encounter with real signs. However, the unstructured questioning by the examiners, a lack of standardization of patients between candidates, and a lack of ability to assess history taking affects the reproducibility and validity of these examinations.

b. *Long case examinations*: During long case examinations, candidates are asked to take a history and perform a complete physical examination on a real patient, frequently chosen from the current in-patient or outpatient cohort. Candidates at different examination sittings may be allocated different patients with varying conditions and clinical signs. Candidates are asked to take a history and perform a complete physical examination in the first 30–45 min, often unobserved by the examiners. Typically, unstructured questioning of the candidates follows this, which is usually focused on their clinical findings, diagnosis and management plan of the patients' problems. The candidates' interaction with the patient, including history taking, general communication and clinical skills is not always observed. Most frequently the discussion is based on the theoretical aspects of the case in question, exploring the depth of candidates' understanding, i.e. their knowledge and the management plan for the patient.

Advantages of Long Cases

a. The use of real patients achieves the highest degree of realism.
b. Ability to assess on rare or complex problems with good clinical signs and symptoms in patients.
c. Ability to choose from a variety of cases. Single case limiting the ability to assess a broad-spectrum of skills.
d. Complete evaluation of the patient's problem—no compartmentalization.

Limitations of Long Cases

1. Inter-case variance or case specificity.
2. Real patient variance or inconsistency in case presentation between candidates.
3. Low inter-rater and intra-rater reliability.
4. High case-specificity.
5. Non-standardized scoring.
6. No blueprinting resulting in random selection of cases for assessment
7. Undue leniency or stringency of the examiners based on the candidate or patient characteristics.

Gleeson has developed OSLER to replace the long case. The reliability and construct validity of the OSLER is better than the long case; which has been achieved by the introduction of different domains to assess the performance of the candidates in each case. But the feasibility of OSLER in undergraduates for indian medical school is questionable because of larger size of students in a class.

In short, the main criticisms of the traditional methods of assessing clinical performance are lack of structure and standardization.

RM Harden (1975) aimed to address the above issues and improve the quality of the assessment of performance by developing OSCE. RM Harden is called the 'Father of OSCE'.

Development of OSCE

Prior to the development of the OSCE, the candidate's assessment could be affected by the patient's performance, examiner bias, a non-standardized marking scheme and the candidate's actual performance. The OSCE was first designed to introduce standardization and reduce the number of variables that could impact the assessment of performance. It comes in the **'show how'** compartment of the Miller's pyramid (Fig. 1).

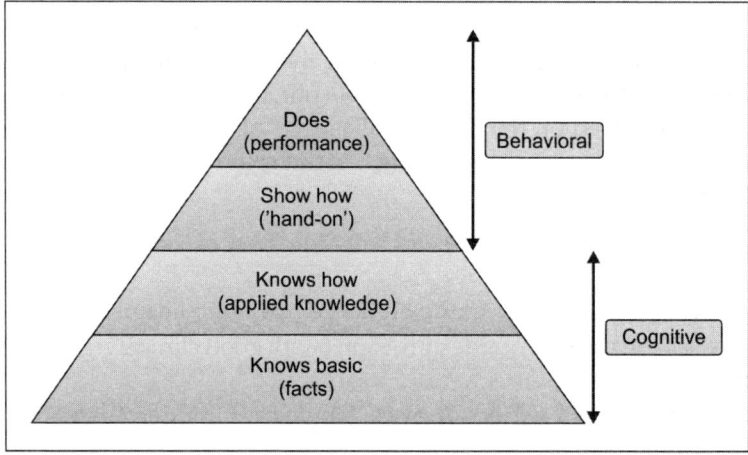

Figure 1: Miller's pyramid

Defining OSCE

A consolidated definition of the OSCE is; "An assessment tool based on the principles of objectivity and standardization, in which the candidates move through a series of time-limited stations in a circuit for the purposes of assessment of professional performance in a simulated environment. At each station, candidates are assessed and marked against standardized scoring rubrics by trained assessors".

Educational Principles of the OSCE

The two major underlying principles of the OSCE are 'objectivity' and 'structure'. Objectivity predominantly depends on standardized scoring rubrics and the same, trained, examiner asking the same questions to every candidate. A well-structured OSCE station on the other hand has a standardized station design assessing a specific clinical task which is blueprinted against the curriculum. A well-designed OSCE has a high level of validity, which in simple terms means that the OSCE assesses what it is designed to assess. At the same time, well-designed OSCE also has been shown to demonstrate a high degree of reliability, i.e. the examination results are reproducible with very little error.

a. **Validity:** High validity.
b. **Reliability:** High reliability.
   Reliability of OSCE also depends on:
   1. The number of stations — 14–18 being optimal
   2. Standardized scoring rubrics.
   3. Using trained examiners.
   4. Standardized patient performance.
c. **Feasibility:** Setting and running an OSCE is very resource intensive in terms of manpower, labor, time, and money; requires very careful organization; and meticulous planning.
d. **Educational impact:** Positive educational impact.

Competencies that can be tested by OSCE/OSPE

OSCE/OSPE can be used to assess a large variety of competencies including skills as well as knowledge in the medical as well as other related fields. Some of the examples include:
- Clinical competencies including history taking, physical examination as well as interpretation of laboratory data.
- Procedural skills including handling of instruments.
- Communication skills including attitude.
- Ethics and many more.

Planning of OSCE/OSPE-Guidelines

1. **Location:** Usually examination should be arranged in the hospital or department with sufficient space to allow ready access to patients. But an area that can be isolated from routine hospital traffic for the duration of the examination is preferable.
2. **Length of examination:** This should depend upon available time and facilities.
3. **Content of each station:** The choice of content must truly represent the defined objectives of the course. Number of stations with 4–5 min at each station. It

has been observed that 4–5 min is a convenient length of time to allow at each station.

   a. *Procedure or performance station*: Perform some task—history taking/examination/test and these are observed by a silent but vigilant examiner and is graded or marked as per checklist and predetermined scheme.

   b. *Response or interpretation station*: Certain questions based on previous station or patient management problems (PMP), MCQ, case history, lab data or ECG.

   c. *Question stations*: Separate stations can be kept as question station where PMP can be asked.

   d. *Rest station*

5. **Designing stations:** Each station must be designed to fit the time available and to measure objectively the skill to be tested.
6. **Selecting patients** for clinical stations
7. **Appointing examiners for clinical stations:** It is important to brief the examiners carefully on their task prior to the day of the test.
8. **Attending to other practical details:** It is necessary to plan these examinations meticulously and includes many minor tasks such as refreshments for examiners and staff, patients and helpers.

Organization of OSCE/OSPE

Requires a lot of thinking and advance planning with time management.

1. Examiners must decide skills to be tested and checklists.
2. Weightage and minimum competency needs to be decided.
3. Patients have to be selected and briefed.
4. Simulated or computer-assisted stations can be included.
5. All staff/observers to be briefed.
6. Organize tables/stations.

Process of OSCE/OSPE

OSCE consists of a series of stations. The candidates rotate through each station in the same sequence. On each station, there is a specific task to perform to evaluate a particular competency. These tasks assess practical, communication, technical, and data interpretation skills and there is a predetermined decision on the competencies to be tested. The performance of a student is evaluated independently on each station, using a standardized checklist. Thus, all students are presented with the same test; and are assessed by the same or equivalent examiners. Students are marked objectively on the checklist by the examiner.

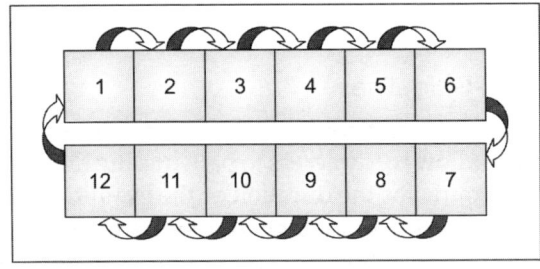

Figure 2: OSCE stations

Advantages of OSCE/OSPE

OSCE/OSPE tests process as well as product. It covers broad area of knowledge/spectrum of skills. The marking is objective. There is increased validity, reliability. There is integration of teaching and evaluation. The variety maintains student interest along with provision of feedback to students and teachers. It provides same standards to all students. Can also evaluate knowledge and attitudes. Large students are covered in limited period.

Challenges of OSCE/OSPE

1. Students are not tested for ability to look patient as a whole as they are tested in compartments.
2. Faculty or observer's fatigue affects adversely.
3. More time, more resources, extensive planning and preparation, team effort and administrative support.

OSCE Variants

a. **Objective-structured practical examination (OSPE):** Assessment of practical skills, knowledge and/or interpretation of data in non-clinical settings.
b. **Objective-structured assessment of technical skills (OSATS):** Designed for objective skills assessment, consisting of a global rating scale and a procedure-specific checklist. It is primarily used for feedback or measuring progress of training in surgical specialties.
c. **Objective-structured video examinations (OSVE):** Videotaped recordings of patient–doctor encounters are shown to students simultaneously and questions related to the video clip are asked. Written answers are marked in a standardized manner.
d. **Team objective-structured clinical examination (TOSCE):** Formative assessment covering common consultations in general practice. A team of students visits each station in a group, performing one task each in a sequence. The candidates are marked for their performance and feedback is provided. The team approach improves efficiency and encourages learning from peers.

Examination Blueprint

Blueprinting is the process of formally determining the content of any examination. In the case of an OSCE, this involves choosing the spread of skills and the frequency with which each appears within an examination. The blueprinting process should ensure that an appropriate sample of the skills-based curriculum is examined and it is mapped to the curriculum, i.e. the examination has adequate content validity.

A blueprint normally consists of a two-dimensional matrix with one axis representing the generic competencies to be tested (e.g. history taking, communication skills, physical examination, management planning, etc.) and the other axis representing the problems or conditions upon which the competencies will be demonstrated.

	History	Examination	Data interpretation
CVS	Infective endocarditis	JVP	ECG
Abdomen	Diarrhea	Palpation of liver	Barium study
RS	Asthma	Chest movements	X-ray
CNS	Development	Neonatal reflexes	CT scan

Choosing a Scoring Rubric and Standard Setting

There are two main types of scoring rubrics—analytical and holistic.

a. Analytical Scoring (Checklist Scale)

A checklist is a list of statements describing the actions expected of the candidates at the station. It is prepared in advance, following consultation with the team designing the OSCE stations and in line with the content and outcomes being assessed.

Sr. no.	Item	Marks	Candidate number				
			1	2	3	4	5
1.	Introduces to the patient and explains procedure to patient	1					
2.	Exposes the arm (uncovers)	0.5					
3.	Places patient's arm across the chest	0.5					
4.	Selects the side at an area just above wrist on lateral side	1					
5.	With gentle pressure, places first three fingers against the radial artery	1					
6.	Counts pulse for one full minute	1					
7.	Tells the pulse rate, rhythm, volume, character	4					
8.	Thanks the patient and covers arm	1					
	Total score	**10**					

b. Holistic Scoring (Global Rating Scale)

Compared with checklists, which are task specific, global rating scales allow the assessor to rate the whole process. Global scales allow examiners to determinant only whether an action was performed, but also how well it was performed. This tool is therefore better for assessing skills where the quality with which it is performed. Hence holistic scales are more useful for assessing areas such as judgment, empathy, organization of knowledge and technical skills. Global ratings are being increasingly used over checklists for marking at OSCE stations, as there is now evidence to suggest that they show greater inter-station reliability, better construct validity, and better concurrent validity compared to checklists.

Example of holistic scoring:

Task: Counseling patient regarding asthma

The student is rated on a scale of 1–5. The examiner score sheet would read as follows:
1. Exceptional
2. Good
3. Average
4. Borderline
5. Poor/Fail

Standard Setting

Standard setting refers to defining the score at which a candidate will pass or fail.
a. **Norm referencing:** The scores have meaning to each other and the pass/fail scores are determined by the relative scores of candidates. Wass, *et al.* (2008) stated that

"Norm-referencing is clearly unacceptable for clinical competency licensing tests, which aim to ensure that candidates are safe to practice."

b. **Criterion referencing:** An absolute clear-cut minimum accepted cut-off is decided beforehand. The specific criterion of passing is predetermined and based on that the decision of certification of competency can be made.

Summary

OSCE by way of direct observation in clinical simulations provides many opportunities for assessment and learning that other traditional evaluation methods also do not offer. The labor- and resource-intensive OSCE has become standard practice in modern assessment of clinical competence, and the results are used for high-stakes decision making at many levels.

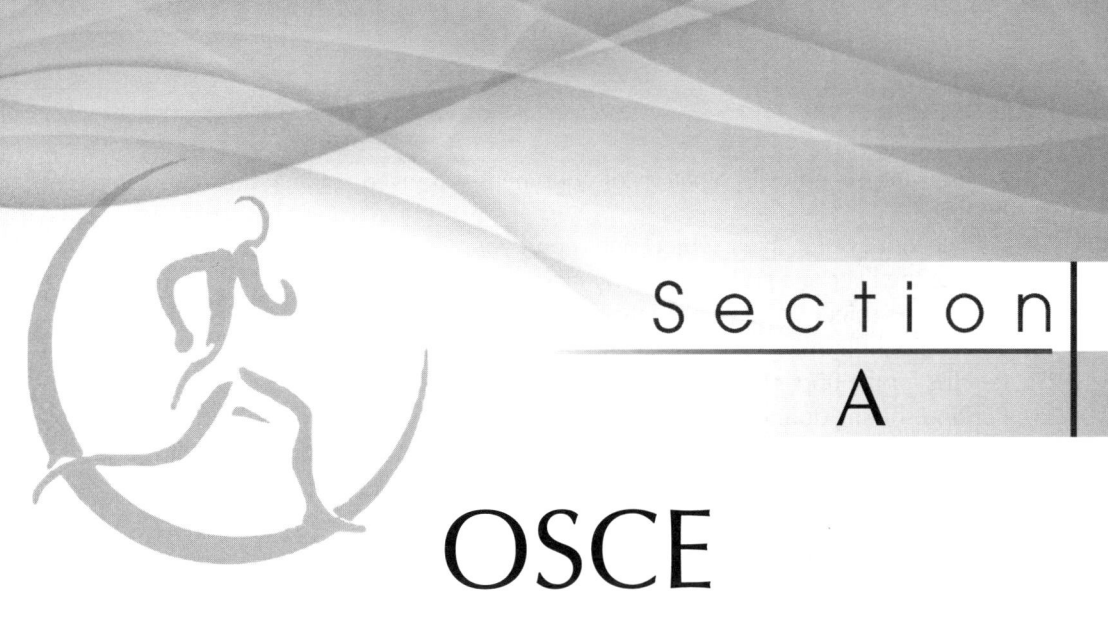

Section

A

OSCE

List of OSCE Stations

OSCE Stations: Respiratory System

1. Perform inspection of chest in lying down position and report your findings
2. Perform palpation of trachea in sitting position and report your findings
3. Palpate the chest for expansion of chest wall and report your findings
4. Elicit tactile vocal fremitus in the given subject and report your findings
5. Auscultate for vocal resonance in the given subject and report your findings
6. Auscultate for breath sounds and report your findings
7. Percuss for the bases of lungs in the given subject and report your findings

OSCE Stations: Cardiovascular System

8. Examine the radial pulse of the given subject and report your findings
9. Examine blood pressure of a given subject in lying down position and report your findings
10. Percuss left border of the heart of a given subject and report your findings
11. Percuss right border of the heart of a given subject and report your findings
12. Auscultate mitral area of the heart of a given subject and report your findings
13. Auscultate tricuspid area of the heart of a given subject and report your findings
14. Auscultate pulmonary area of the heart of a given subject and report your findings
15. Auscultate aortic area of the heart of a given subject and report your findings
16. Palpate apex beat in given subject and report your findings
17. Inspect precordium of a given subject in lying down position and report your findings
18. Record JVP in a given subject and report your findings
19. Auscultate for the 1st heart sound in the given subject and report your findings
20. Auscultate for the 2nd heart sound in the given subject and report your findings

OSCE Stations: Abdomen

21. Inspect the abdomen of a given subject in lying down position and report your findings

22. Perform the superficial palpation of abdomen of a given subject and report your findings.
23. Palpate kidney of a given subject and report your findings
24. Palpate the liver of a given subject by classical method and report your findings
25. Palpate the spleen of a given subject by classical method and report your findings
26. Elicit fluid thrill in a given subject and report your findings
27. Percuss for the upper border of liver and report your findings
28. Perform shifting dullness in a given subject and report your findings
29. Perform horseshoe-shaped dullness in a given subject and report your findings
30. Auscultate for the abdominal sounds in a given subject and report your findings

OSCE Stations: CNS: Cranial Nerves

31. Examine I cranial nerve of a given subject and report your findings
32. Examine II cranial nerve of a given subject for color vision and report your findings
33a. Examine III, IV, VI cranial nerves of a given subject for movement of eyeball and report your findings
33b. Examine III cranial nerve of a given subject for light reflex and report your findings
33c. Examine III cranial nerve of a given subject for accommodation reflex and report your findings
34. Examine V cranial nerve of a given subject and report your findings
35. Examine VII cranial nerve of a given subject and report your findings
36. Perform Rinne's test in a given subject and report your findings
37. Examine X cranial nerve in a given subject and report your findings
38a. Examine XI cranial nerve in a given subject and report your findings
38b. Examine XII cranial nerve in a given subject and report your findings
39. Perform confrontation test in the given subject and report your findings

OSCE Stations: CNS: Motor System

40. Examine for power of muscle in upper extremity of a given subject and report your findings
41. Examine for power of muscle in lower extremity of a given subject and report your findings
42. Examine for co-ordination in upper limb of a given subject and report your findings
43. Examine for co-ordination in lower limb of a given subject and report your findings
44. Assess the tone of flexors for upper limb elbow joint of a given subject and report your findings
45. Assess the tone of a muscle in lower limb knee joint of a given subject and report your findings.

OSCE Stations: CNS: Reflexes

46. Elicit biceps jerk in a given subject in sitting position and report your findings
47. Elicit biceps jerk in a given subject in spine position and report your findings
48a. Elicit triceps jerk in a given subject in sitting position and report your findings
48b. Elicit triceps jerk in a given subject in supine position and report your findings
49a. Elicit knee jerk in a given subject in sitting position and report your findings
49b. Elicit knee jerk in a given subject in spine position and report your findings

50a. Elicit ankle jerk in a given subject in sitting position and report your findings
50b. Elicit ankle jerk in a given subject in supine position and report your findings
51. Elicit plantar reflex in a given subject and report your findings
52. Elicit abdominal reflex in a given subject and report your findings
53. Elicit supinator jerk in a given subject and report your findings
54. Elicit jaw jerk in a given subject and report your findings

OSCE Stations: CNS: Sensory System

55. Examine the given subject for fine touch on forearm anterior aspect and report your findings
56. Examine the given subject for tactile localization on forearm anterior aspect and report your findings
57. Examine the given subject for sensation of pressure on forearm anterior aspect and report your findings
58. Examine the given subject for two-point discrimination on forearm anterior aspect and report your findings
59. Examine the given subject for sense of temperature on forearm anterior aspect and report your findings
60. Examine the given subject for sense of position and movement in upper limbs and report your findings
61. Examine the given subject for vibration sense and report your findings
62. Examine the given subject for sense of superficial pain on forearm anterior aspect and report your findings
63. Examine the given subject for sense of deep pain and report your findings
64. Examine the given subject for sense of stereognosis and report your findings

Respiratory System

Respiratory System: Date:

Station no. 1: Perform inspection of chest in lying down position and report your findings.

Domains tested: Psychomotor, affective and communication

S. no.	Steps	Marks	R. no. 1	R. no. 2	R. no. 3
A.	**Checklist**				
1.	Stands on the right side of the subject	1			
2.	Explains the procedure in local language	1			
3.	Exposes the chest properly	1			
4.	Inspects for the size, shape and type of breathing from foot end	1.5			
5.	Inspects for the size, shape and type of breathing from side	1.5			
6.	Counts the rate of respiration for 1 min by observing the up and down movement of chest	1			
7.	Covers the exposed area properly	1			
8.	Looks for the scar, visible veins, any swelling, apex impulse	2			
9.	Narrates the findings to the observer Size, shape, type of breathing Rate of respiration Scars, visible veins, any swelling Apex impulse	4			
B.	**Assessment of Professional Behavior**				
1.	Informs subject regarding completion of procedure and thanks the subject	1			
	Total Marks	**15**			
	Correction Factor				
	Final Score				
	Global Rating: 1. Poor; 2. Unsatisfactory; 3. Satisfactory; 4. Good; 5. Excellent				
Observer's Comment (based on general observation):					
Signature of Observer					

Response stations:
1. Enumerate the muscles involved in quiet inspiration
2. Enumerate the accessory muscles of respiration.
3. Write the formula for dyspneic index.

Respiratory System: Date:

Station no. 2: Perform palpation of trachea in sitting position and report your findings.

Domains tested: Psychomotor, affective and communication

S. no.	Steps	Marks	R. no. 1	R. no. 2	R. no. 3
A.	**Checklist**				
1.	Stands on the right side of the subject	1			
2.	Explains the procedure in local language	1			
3.	Gives the correct position to the subject needed for the examination (sitting position)	1			
4.	Asks the subject to semi-flex the head	1			
5.	Places the tip of the index and ring fingers on the right and left sternal ends of the clavicle, respectively and middle finger just above the sternal notch	2			
6.	Palpates the tracheal ring by pushing forward the middle finger	2			
7.	Feels for the space between the trachea and the sternocleidomastoid muscle with the middle finger on both sides	2			
8.	Narrates the findings to the observer	2			
B.	**Assessment of Professional Behavior**				
1.	Informs subject regarding completion of procedure and thanks the subject	1			
	Total Marks	**13**			
	Correction Factor				
	Final Score				
	Global Rating: 1. Poor; 2. Unsatisfactory; 3. Satisfactory; 4. Good; 5. Excellent				
Observer's Comment (based on general observation):					
Signature of Observer					

Response stations:

1. On examination, trachea was found to be shifted on left. Enumerate any two causes of shifting of trachea on the side of the lung lesion and away from the side of the lung lesion.
2. Trail sign is the palpation method to detect the shifting of trachea: TRUE or FALSE.

Respiratory System: Date:

Station no. 3: Palpate the chest for expansion of chest wall and report your findings.

Domains tested: Psychomotor, affective and communication

S. no.	Steps	Marks	R. no. 1	R. no. 2	R. no. 3
A.	**Checklist**				
1.	Stands on the right side of the subject	1			
2.	Explains the procedure in the local language	1			
3.	Rubs the palms together	1			
4.	Asks the subject to take deep breaths	1			
5.	Places the palms on both sides of chest wall with the thumbs approximated in the centre	2			
6.	Checks for the displacement of the thumb on both sides from the midline during inspiration	2			
7.	Palpates upper, middle and lower lobes anteriorly and posteriorly	6			
8.	Narrates the findings to the observer	2			
B.	**Assessment of Professional Behavior**				
1.	Informs subject regarding completion of procedure and thanks the subject	1			
	Total Marks	**17**			
	Correction Factor				
	Final Score				
	Global Rating: 1. Poor; 2. Unsatisfactory; 3. Satisfactory; 4. Good; 5. Excellent				
Observer's Comment (based on general observation):					
Signature of Observer					

Response stations:

1. Enumerate any three abnormal types of chest wall.
2. The movement on right side of chest wall is decreased as compared to left side. Enumerate any two causes of reduced expansion on right side.

Respiratory System: Date:

Station no. 4: Elicit tactile vocal fremitus in the given subject and report your findings.

Domains tested: Psychomotor, affective and communication

S. no.	Steps	Marks	R. no. 1	R. no. 2	R. no. 3
A.	**Checklist**				
1.	Stands on the right side of the subject	1			
2.	Explains the procedure in the local language	1			
3.	Rubs the palms together	1			
4.	Asks the subject to say 1, 2, 3 in their local language	1			
5.	Places the ulnar border of right hand on intercostal spaces	1			
6.	Elicits tactile vocal fremitus from second intercostal space downwards and examines				
	Anteriorly (bilaterally)	2			
	Axillary (bilaterally)	2			
	Posteriorly (bilaterally)	2			
7.	Narrates the findings to the observer	2			
B.	**Assessment of Professional Behavior**				
1.	Informs subject regarding completion of procedure and thanks the subject	1			
	Total Marks	**14**			
	Correction Factor				
	Final Score				
	Global Rating: 1. Poor; 2. Unsatisfactory; 3. Satisfactory; 4. Good; 5. Excellent				
Observer's Comment (based on general observation):					
Signature of Observer					

Response stations:

1. Define tactile vocal fremitus.
2. Enumerate two causes of increased tactile vocal fremitus.

Respiratory System: Date:

Station no. 5: Auscultate for vocal resonance in the given subject and report your findings.

Domains tested: Psychomotor, affective and communication

S. no.	Steps	Marks	R. no. 1	R. no. 2	R. no. 3
A.	**Checklist**				
1.	Stands on the right side of the subject	1			
2.	Explains the procedure in the local language	1			
3.	Holds the stethoscope with earpiece pointing forwards and medially	1			
4.	Checks whether the stethoscope is on; from the side of diaphragm	1			
5.	Asks the subject to say 1, 2, 3 in their local language	1			
6.	Auscultates in the following areas: Supraclavicular, infraclavicular (bilaterally)	2			
	Anterior chest wall (bilaterally)	2			
	Axillary (bilaterally)	2			
	Posterior chest wall—suprascapular, interscapular, infrascapular (bilaterally)	2			
7.	Narrates the findings to the observer	2			
B.	**Assessment of Professional Behavior**				
1.	Informs subject regarding completion of procedure and thanks the subject	1			
	Total Marks	**16**			
	Correction Factor				
	Final Score				
	Global Rating: 1. Poor; 2. Unsatisfactory; 3. Satisfactory; 4. Good; 5. Excellent				
Observer's Comment (based on general observation):					
Signature of Observer					

Response stations:

1. Enumerate two causes of increased vocal resonance.
2. Define whispering pectoriloquy.

Respiratory System: Date:

Station no. 6: Auscultate for breath sounds of given subject and report your findings.

Domains tested: Psychomotor, affective and communication

S. no.	Steps	Marks	R. no. 1	R. no. 2	R. no. 3
A.	**Checklist**				
1.	Stands on the right side of the subject	1			
2.	Orients the patient about the procedure in local language	2			
3.	Asks the subject to expose the part to be examined and covers the rest of the body with a sheet	1			
4.	Holds the stethoscope with its earpiece pointing forwards and medially	1			
5.	Checks whether the stethoscope is on; from the side of diaphragm	1			
6.	Asks the subject to take deep breaths	1			
7.	Auscultates over the; Trachea All over the chest wall anteriorly and posteriorly Axillary and infra-axillary Suprascapular and infrascapular	5			
8.	Narrates the findings to the observer	2			
B.	**Assessment of Professional Behavior**				
1.	Informs subject regarding completion of procedure and thanks the subject	1			
	Total Marks	**15**			
	Correction Factor				
	Final Score				
	Global Rating: 1. Poor; 2. Unsatisfactory; 3. Satisfactory; 4. Good; 5. Excellent				
Observer's Comment (based on general observation):					
Signature of Observer					

Response stations:

1. Differentiate between vesicular and bronchial breath sounds (any 3 points).
2. Enumerate any two causes of bronchial breath sounds over chest.

Respiratory System: Date:

Station no. 7: Percuss for the bases of lungs in the given subject and report your findings.

Domains tested: Psychomotor, affective and communication

S. no.	Steps	Marks	R. no. 1	R. no. 2	R. no. 3
A.	**Checklist**				
1.	Stands on the right side of the subject	1			
2.	Orients the patient about the procedure in local language	2			
3.	Asks the subject to expose the part to be examined and covers the rest of the body with a sheet	1			
4.	Places the pleximeter finger parallel to the intercostal muscle and taps its middle phalanx with middle finger of right hand in perpendicular direction	1			
5.	Carries out the percussion movement by flexion and extension at the wrist joint	1			
6.	Starts percussing from 2nd intercostal space and compares with opposite side of chest wall.	1			
7.	Goes up to 6th intercostal space in anterior mammillary line and 7th intercostal space in mid-axillary line	5			
8.	Percusses posteriorly on scapular and infrascapular area	2			
9.	Narrates the findings to the observer	1			
B.	**Assessment of Professional Behavior**				
1.	Informs subject regarding completion of procedure and thanks the subject	1			
	Total Marks	**16**			
	Correction Factor				
	Final Score				
	Global Rating: 1. Poor; 2. Unsatisfactory; 3. Satisfactory; 4. Good; 5. Excellent				
Observer's Comment (based on general observation):					
Signature of Observer					

Response stations:

1. Enumerate one cause each for resonant note, hyperresonant note, dull note and stony dull note in percussion.
2. Percussion should be carried from resonant to dull note. TRUE or FALSE.

Cardiovascular System

Cardiovascular System: Date:

Station no. 8: Examine the radial pulse of the given subject and report your findings.

Domains tested: Psychomotor, affective and communication

S. no.	Steps	Marks	R. no. 1	R. no. 2	R. no. 3
A.	**Checklist**				
1.	Stands on the right side of the subject	1			
2.	Explains the procedure in the local language	1			
3.	Rubs the palm before procedure	2			
4.	Positions hand as pronated forearm and slightly flexed wrist	1			
5.	Places the three fingers over the radial pulse properly (index, middle and ring fingers in ascending order)	2			
6.	Counts the pulse for 1 minute	2			
7.	Examines pulse of opposite side	1			
8.	Mentions the findings: Rate, rhythm, volume, characteristic, condition of vessel wall and equality on both sides	6			
9.	Narrates the findings to the observer	1			
B.	**Assessment of Professional Behavior**				
1.	Informs subject regarding completion of procedure and thanks the subject	1			
	Total Marks	**18**			
	Correction Factor				
	Final Score				
	Global Rating: 1. Poor; 2. Unsatisfactory; 3. Satisfactory; 4. Good; 5. Excellent				
Observer's Comment (based on general observation):					
Signature of Observer					

Response stations:

1. Define apex-pulse deficit. Enumerate any one cause of it.
2. Enumerate any one cause of radiofemoral delay.
3. Draw a labeled diagram of pulse wave.
4. Give two abnormal forms or characters of the arterial pulse.

Cardiovascular System: Date:

Station no. 9: Examine blood pressure of a given subject in lying down position and report your findings.

Domains tested: Psychomotor, affective and communication

S. no.	Steps	Marks	R. no. 1	R. no. 2	R. no. 3
A.	**Checklist**				
1.	Stands on the right side of the subject	1			
2.	Makes subject comfortable in lying down position	1			
3.	Explains the procedure in the local language	1			
4.	Exposes the arm of the subject properly	1			
5.	Ties the BP cuff properly at the level of the heart	2			
6.	Checks for the zero reading on mercury manometer	1			
7.	Records SBP (systolic blood pressure) by palpatory method	2			
8.	Places the chestpiece of the stethoscope on the brachial artery	2			
9.	Inflates the pressure cuff above systolic blood pressure	2			
10.	Deflates the cuff slowly	2			
11.	Removes the cuff and places it properly in the sphygmomanometer	2			
12.	Narrates the findings to the observer	2			
13.	Covers the exposed area properly	1			
B.	**Assessment of Professional Behavior**				
1.	Informs subject regarding completion of procedure and thanks the subject	1			
	Total Marks	**21**			
	Correction Factor				
	Final Score				
	Global Rating: 1. Poor; 2. Unsatisfactory; 3. Satisfactory; 4. Good; 5. Excellent				
	Observer's Comment (based on general observation):				
	Signature of Observer				

Response stations:

1. Enumerate the mean blood pressure range of working of baroreceptors.
2. The chemoreceptors respond to the oxygen dissolved in the blood. TRUE or FALSE.
3. Define essential hypertension. Enumerate any two causes of essential hypertension.

Cardiovascular System: Date:

Station no. 10: Percuss left border of the heart of a given subject and report your findings.

Domains tested: Psychomotor, affective and communication

S. no.	Steps	Marks	R. no. 1	R. no. 2	R. no. 3
A.	**Checklist**				
1.	Stands on the right side of the subject	1			
2.	Explains detail procedure and takes consent	1			
3.	Exposes the precordium	1			
4.	Counts from the second intercostal space and locates 5th ICS on left side	2			
5.	Starts percussing from 5th intercoastal space lateral to medial on left side	2			
6.	Percusses upwards in the same manner till second intercoastal space on left side.	2			
7.	Narrates the findings to the observer	2			
8.	Covers the exposed area properly	1			
B.	**Assessment of Professional Behavior**				
1.	Informs subject regarding completion of procedure and thanks the subject	1			
	Total Marks	**13**			
	Correction Factor				
	Final Score				
	Global Rating: 1. Poor; 2. Unsatisfactory; 3. Satisfactory; 4. Good; 5. Excellent				
Observer's Comment (based on general observation):					
Signature of Observer					

Response stations:

1. Enumerate the two structures forming the left heart border.
2. Enumerate the conditions that can be diagnosed using percussion of left heart border.

Cardiovascular System:
Date:

Station no. 11: Percuss right border of the heart of a given subject and report your findings.

Domains tested: Psychomotor, affective and communication

S. no.	Steps	Marks	R. no. 1	R. no. 2	R. no. 3
A.	**Checklist**				
1.	Stands on the right side of the subject	1			
2.	Explains detail procedure and takes consent	1			
3.	Exposes the right side of chest wall	1			
4.	Percusses from the second intercostal space down in the mid-clavicular line and locates the upper border of liver dullness	2			
5.	Shifts the percussing finger one space above	2			
6.	Percusses from lateral aspect towards the sternum	2			
7.	Repeats the percussion from lateral aspect towards sternum in 4th and 3rd intercostal space	2			
8.	Narrates the findings to the observer	2			
B.	**Assessment of Professional Behavior**				
1.	Informs subject regarding completion of procedure and thanks the subject	1			
	Total Marks	**14**			
	Correction Factor				
	Final Score				
	Global Rating: 1. Poor; 2. Unsatisfactory; 3. Satisfactory; 4. Good; 5. Excellent				
Observer's Comment (based on general observation):					
Signature of Observer					

Response stations:
1. Enumerate the two structures forming the right heart border.
2. Enumerate the conditions that can be diagnosed using percussion of right heart border.

Cardiovascular System: Date:

Station no. 12: Auscultate mitral area of the heart of a given subject and report your findings.

Domains tested: Psychomotor, affective and communication

S. no.	Steps	Marks	R. no. 1	R. no. 2	R. no. 3
A.	**Checklist**				
1.	Stands on the right side of the subject	1			
2.	Explains the procedure in the local language	1			
3.	Exposes the precordium	1			
4.	Counts the intercostal spaces	1			
5.	Locates the mitral area and pin points with index finger over that area	2			
6.	Holds the stethoscope with its earpiece pointing forwards and medially	1			
7.	Checks whether the stethoscope is on; from the side of diaphragm	1			
8.	Auscultates heart sounds for one minute	2			
9.	Correlates with the carotid pulsation	2			
10.	Narrates the findings to the observer	2			
11.	Covers the exposed area properly	1			
B.	**Assessment of Professional Behavior**				
1.	Informs subject regarding completion of procedure and thanks the subject	1			
	Total Marks	**16**			
	Correction Factor				
	Final Score				
	Global Rating: 1. Poor; 2. Unsatisfactory; 3. Satisfactory; 4. Good; 5. Excellent				
Observer's Comment (based on general observation):					
Signature of Observer					

Response stations:
1. Differentiate between 1st and 2nd heart sounds
2. Mention cause of 1st and 2nd heart sounds.

Cardiovascular System: Date:

Station no. 13: Auscultate tricuspid area of the heart of a given subject and report your findings.

Domains tested: Psychomotor, affective and communication

S. no.	Steps	Marks	R. no. 1	R. no. 2	R. no. 3
A.	**Checklist**				
1.	Stands on the right side of the subject	1			
2.	Explains the procedure in the local language	1			
3.	Exposes the precordium	1			
4.	Counts the intercostal spaces on left side	2			
5.	Locates the tricuspid area in 5th intercoastal space lateral to the sternal border	2			
6.	Holds the stethoscope with its earpiece pointing forwards and medially.	1			
7.	Checks whether the stethoscope is on; from the side of diaphragm	1			
8.	Auscultates the heart sounds for complete one minute	1			
9.	Correlates with the carotid pulsation	2			
10.	Narrates the findings to the observer	1			
11.	Covers the exposed area properly	1			
B.	**Assessment of Professional Behavior**				
1.	Informs subject regarding completion of procedure and thanks the subject	1			
	Total Marks	**15**			
	Correction Factor				
	Final Score				
	Global Rating: 1. Poor; 2. Unsatisfactory; 3. Satisfactory; 4. Good; 5. Excellent				
Observer's Comment (based on general observation):					
Signature of Observer					

Response stations:
1. Differentiate between 1st and 2nd heart sounds
2. Mention cause of 1st and 2nd heart sounds.

Cardiovascular System: Date:

Station no. 14: Auscultate pulmonary area of the heart of a given subject and report your findings.

Domains tested: Psychomotor, affective and communication

S. no.	Steps	Marks	R. no. 1	R. no. 2	R. no. 3
A.	**Checklist**				
1.	Stands on the right side of the subject	1			
2.	Explains the procedure in the local language	1			
3.	Exposes the precordium	1			
4.	Counts the 2nd intercostal space on left side	2			
5.	Locates the pulmonary area at 2 cm away from the sternal border	2			
6.	Holds the stethoscope with its earpiece pointing forwards and medially.	1			
7.	Checks whether the stethoscope is on; from the side of diaphragm	1			
8.	Correlates with the carotid pulsation	2			
9.	Narrates the findings to the observer	2			
10.	Covers the exposed area properly	1			
B.	**Assessment of Professional Behavior**				
1.	Informs subject regarding completion of procedure and thanks the subject	1			
	Total Marks	**15**			
	Correction Factor				
	Final Score				
	Global Rating: 1. Poor; 2. Unsatisfactory; 3. Satisfactory; 4. Good; 5. Excellent				
Observer's Comment (based on general observation):					
Signature of Observer					

Response stations:

1. Differentiate between 1st and 2nd heart sounds
2. Mention cause of 1st and 2nd heart sounds.

Cardiovascular System: Date:

Station no. 15: Auscultate aortic area of the heart of a given subject and report your findings.

Domains tested: Psychomotor, affective and communication

S. no.	Steps	Marks	R. no. 1	R. no. 2	R. no. 3
A.	**Checklist**				
1.	Stands on the right side of the subject	1			
2.	Explains the procedure in the local language	1			
3.	Exposes the precordium	1			
4.	Counts the intercostal spaces on right side	2			
5.	Locates the aortic area and pinpoints with index finger over that area	2			
6.	Holds the stethoscope with its earpiece pointing forwards and medially	1			
7.	Checks whether the stethoscope is on; from the side of diaphragm	1			
8.	Auscultates the heart sounds for complete one minute	1			
9.	Correlates with the carotid pulsation	2			
10.	Narrates the findings to the observer	2			
11.	Covers the exposed area properly	1			
B.	**Assessment of Professional Behavior**				
1.	Informs subject regarding completion of procedure and thanks the subject	1			
	Total Marks	**16**			
	Correction factor				
	Final Score				
	Global Rating: 1. Poor; 2. Unsatisfactory; 3. Satisfactory; 4. Good; 5. Excellent				
Observer's Comment (based on general observation):					
Signature of Observer					

Response stations:
1. Differentiate between 1st and 2nd heart sounds
2. Mention cause of 1st and 2nd heart sounds.

Cardiovascular System: Date:

Station no. 16: Palpate apex beat in given subject and report your findings.

Domains tested: Psychomotor, affective and communication

S. no.	Steps	Marks	R. no. 1	R. no. 2	R. no. 3
A.	**Checklist**				
1.	Stands on the right side of the subject	1			
2.	Orients the patient about the procedure in local language	1			
3.	Asks the subject to expose the part to be examined and covers the rest of the body with a sheet	1			
4.	Rubs the palms together	1			
5.	Inspects for any visible apical impulse over the precordium	1			
6.	Keeps his right palm over the apical impulse/over the left precordium	2			
7.	Feels for the same impulse with the ulnar border of his right hand	2			
8.	Localizes the apex impulse with the tip of the right index finger	2			
9.	Locates the situation of apex beat by counting the intercostal spaces	2			
10.	Narrates the findings to the observer	1			
11.	Covers the exposed area properly	1			
B.	**Assessment of Professional Behavior**				
1.	Informs subject regarding completion of procedure and thanks the subject	1			
	Total Marks	**16**			
	Correction Factor				
	Final Score				
	Global Rating: 1. Poor; 2. Unsatisfactory; 3. Satisfactory; 4. Good; 5. Excellent				
Observer's Comment (based on general observation):					
Signature of Observer					

Response stations:

1. Define apex beat.
2. Write causes of shifting of apex beat to right side.

Cardiovascular System: Date:

Station no. 17: Inspect precordium of a given subject in lying down position and report your findings.

Domains tested: Psychomotor, affective and communication

S. no.	Steps	Marks	R. no. 1	R. no. 2	R. no. 3
A.	**Checklist**				
1.	Stands on the right side of the subject	1			
2.	Explains detail procedure and obtains verbal consent	1			
3.	Exposes the precordium, i.e. anterior aspect of chest wall	1			
4.	Inspects for dyspnea, cyanosis, shape of chest, neck veins, veins of chest wall, cardiac impulse and other pulsation on chest and reports the findings	6			
5.	Covers the exposed area properly	1			
B.	**Assessment of Professional Behavior**				
1.	Informs subject regarding completion of procedure and thanks the subject	1			
	Total Marks	**11**			
	Correction Factor				
	Final Score				
	Global Rating: 1. Poor; 2. Unsatisfactory; 3. Satisfactory; 4. Good; 5. Excellent				
Observer's Comment (based on general observation):					
Signature of Observer					

Response stations:
1. Enumerate four properties of cardiac muscle.
2. Enumerate the pacemaker tissues of the heart.
3. Enumerate any two metabolic properties of heart.
4. Enumerate any four mechanical properties of cardiac muscle.
5. List the unipolar recording leads in an ECG.

Cardiovascular System: Date:

Station no. 18: Record JVP in a given subject and report your findings.

Domains tested: Psychomotor, affective and communication

S. no.	Steps	Marks	R. no. 1	R. no. 2	R. no. 3
A.	**Checklist**				
1.	Stands on the right side of the subject	1			
2.	Explains detail procedure and takes verbal consent	1			
3.	Exposes the neck area and chest	1			
4.	Observes the jugular vein in the neck in lying down position	1			
5.	Raises the head along with shoulder of the subject to 30–45°	1			
6.	Locates the uppermost part of the jugular vein where it is still distended	1			
7.	Identifies the sternal angle and keeps the ruler on sternal angle in vertical direction	2			
8.	Draws imaginary horizontal line from the uppermost distended part of the jugular vein up to the sternal angle (ruler)	5			
9.	Measures the height (from sternum to the imaginary line drawn from jugular vein)	3			
10.	Narrates the findings to the observer	2			
11.	Covers the exposed area properly	1			
B.	**Assessment of Professional Behavior**				
1.	Informs subject regarding completion of procedure and thanks the subject	1			
	Total Marks	**20**			
	Correction Factor				
	Final Score				
	Global Rating: 1. Poor; 2. Unsatisfactory; 3. Satisfactory; 4. Good; 5. Excellent				
Observer's Comment (based on general observation):					
Signature of Observer					

Response stations:

1. Enumerate various waves of JVP.
2. Enumerate the various events in cardiac cycle.
3. Enumerate the various events in ventricular systole of the cardiac cycle.
4. Mention the systolic peak pressure in left ventricle and right ventricle.

Cardiovascular System: Date:

Station no. 19: Auscultate for the 1st heart sound in the given subject and report your findings.

Domains tested: Psychomotor, affective and communication

S. no.	Steps	Marks	R. no. 1	R. no. 2	R. no. 3
A.	**Checklist**				
1.	Stands on the right side of the subject	1			
2.	Explains detail procedure and takes verbal consent	1			
3.	Checks for the normal functioning of the stethoscope	2			
4.	Exposes the complete chest of the subject	1			
5.	Locates the mitral area, first by identifying the 2nd intercostal space on left side and then going down by counting the intercostal spaces to 5th intercostal space in midclavicular line	4			
6.	Places the diaphragm of the stethoscope on the identified mitral area	1			
7.	Places the earpiece of stethoscope comfortably into the ears along the direction of the ear canals	1			
8.	Palpates the external carotid artery by another hand to identify 1st heart sound	3			
9.	Listens to the heart sound for one minute and reports findings	2			
10.	Covers the exposed area properly	1			
B.	**Assessment of Professional Behavior**				
1.	Informs subject regarding completion of procedure and thanks the subject	1			
	Total Marks	**18**			
	Correction Factor				
	Final Score				
	Global Rating: 1. Poor; 2. Unsatisfactory; 3. Satisfactory; 4. Good; 5. Excellent				
Observer's Comment (based on general observation):					
Signature of Observer					

Cardiovascular System: Date:

Station no. 20: Auscultate for the 2nd heart sound in the given subject and report your findings.

Domains tested: Psychomotor, affective and communication

S. no.	Steps	Marks	R. no. 1	R. no. 2	R. no. 3
A.	**Checklist**				
1.	Stands on the right side of the subject	1			
2.	Explains detail procedure and takes verbal consent	1			
3.	Checks for the normal functioning of the stethoscope	1			
4.	Exposes the complete chest of the subject	1			
5.	Locates the tricuspid area, located on left lower sternal border in 4th intercostal space	3			
6.	Places the diaphragm of the stethoscope on the identified tricuspid area	2			
7.	Places the earpiece of stethoscope comfortably into the ears along the direction of the ear canals	2			
8.	Palpates the external carotid artery by another hand to identify 2nd heart sound	3			
9.	Listens to the heart sound for one minute and reports findings	2			
10.	Covers the exposed area properly	1			
B.	**Assessment of Professional Behavior**				
1.	Informs subject regarding completion of procedure and thanks the subject	1			
	Total Marks	**18**			
	Correction Factor				
	Final Score				
	Global Rating: 1. Poor; 2. Unsatisfactory; 3. Satisfactory; 4. Good; 5. Excellent				
Observer's Comment (based on general observation):					
Signature of Observer					

Response stations:

1. List any two differences between semilunar and tricuspid valves.
2. List any two differences between 1st and 2nd heart sounds.
3. Enumerate the causes of first and second heart sounds.
4. Define pacemaker potential.
5. Define idioventricular rhythm.
6. State Frank-Starling law.
7. Draw a well-labeled diagram of pressure changes in the left side of the heart during the cardiac cycle.

8. Draw a well-labeled diagram of volume changes in the left side of the heart during the cardiac cycle.
9. Draw a well-labeled diagram of ECG changes in the left side of the heart during the cardiac cycle.
10. Enumerate the various events in cardiac cycle.
11. Enumerate the various events in ventricular systole of the cardiac cycle.
12. Mention the systolic peak pressure in left ventricle and right ventricle.

Abdomen

Abdomen: Date:

Station no. 21: Inspect the abdomen of a given subject in lying down position and report your findings.

Domains tested: Psychomotor, affective and communication

S. no.	Steps	Marks	R. no. 1	R. no. 2	R. no. 3
A.	**Checklist**				
1.	Stands on the right side of the subject	1			
2.	Explains detail procedure and takes verbal consent	1			
3.	Exposes the abdomen fully up to just above the xiphisternum	1			
4.	Inspects for shape of abdomen, umbilicus, movement of abdominal wall, presence of any visible pulsations, skin of abdomen, any prominent veins, etc. and report your findings	6			
5.	Covers the exposed area properly.	1			
B.	**Assessment of Professional Behavior**				
1.	Informs subject regarding completion of procedure and thanks the subject	1			
	Total Marks	**11**			
	Correction Factor				
	Final Score				
	Global Rating: 1. Poor; 2. Unsatisfactory; 3. Satisfactory; 4. Good; 5. Excellent				
Observer's Comment (based on general observation):					
Signature of Observer					

Response stations:
1. Draw a diagram of showing nine arbitrary divisions of abdomen.
2. Differentiate between myenteric and Meissener's plexus.
3. Draw and label cross-section of GIT showing different layers of its wall and structure of a villus.
4. Draw a well-labeled diagram of physiological anatomy of stomach.
5. Differentiate between extrinsic and intrinsic innervation of GIT.

Abdomen: Date:

Station no. 22: Perform the superficial palpation of abdomen of a given subject and report your findings.

Domains tested: Psychomotor, affective and communication

S. no.	Steps	Marks	R. no. 1	R. no. 2	R. no. 3
A.	**Checklist**				
1.	Stands on the right side of the subject	1			
2.	Explains detail procedure and takes verbal consent	1			
3.	Exposes the abdomen fully up to just above the xiphisternum	1			
4.	Rubs the palm against each other to warm	2			
5.	Starts palpating superficially from left iliac region, goes anticlockwise to end in the suprapubic region	4			
6.	Notes for any swelling or tumour mass, tenderness or rigidity and report your findings	3			
7.	Covers the exposed area properly	1			
B.	**Assessment of Professional Behavior**				
1.	Informs subject regarding completion of procedure and thanks the subject	1			
	Total Marks	**14**			
	Correction Factor				
	Final Score				
	Global Rating: 1. Poor; 2. Unsatisfactory; 3. Satisfactory; 4. Good; 5. Excellent				
Observer's Comment (based on general observation):					
Signature of Observer					

Response stations:
1. Differentiate between myenteric and Meissener's plexus.
2. Define deglutition and enumerate various stages of deglutition.
3. Write down the pathway for defecation reflex.
4. Differentiate between extrinsic and intrinsic innervation of GIT.

Abdomen: Date:

Station no. 23: Palpate kidney of a given subject and report your findings.

Domains tested: Psychomotor, affective and communication

S. no.	Steps	Marks	R. no. 1	R. no. 2	R. no. 3
A.	**Checklist**				
1.	Stands on the right side of the subject	1			
2.	Explains detail procedure and takes verbal consent	1			
3.	Exposes the abdomen fully up to just above the xiphisternum	1			
4.	Ensures that his own hands are warm	1			
5.	Asks the subject to breath quietly	1			
6.	Places the right hand anteriorly in the right lumbar region (for left kidney) while the left hand is placed posteriorly in the loin	4			
7.	Asks the subject to take deep breath in, presses the left hand forwards and the right hand upwards and inwards	2			
8.	Repeats the same procedure for right kidney	6			
9.	Narrates the findings to the observer	1			
10.	Covers the exposed area properly	1			
B.	**Assessment of Professional Behavior**				
1.	Informs subject regarding completion of procedure and thanks the subject	1			
	Total Marks	**20**			
	Correction Factor				
	Final Score				
	Global Rating: 1. Poor; 2. Unsatisfactory; 3. Satisfactory; 4. Good; 5. Excellent				
Observer's Comment (based on general observation):					
Signature of Observer					

Response stations:
1. Enumerate kidney function tests
2. Write two non-excretory functions of kidney
3. Enumerate any four factors affecting glomerular filtration rate.
4. Enumerate four conditions of acid-base imbalance.
5. Enlist any four functions of kidney.
6. Enumerate the factors affecting GFR.
7. Write four peculiarities of renal blood flow.
8. Write two features of juxtaglomerular apparatus.
9. Enumerate two sources of renal blood flow.
10. Name two layers of glomerular capillary wall.
11. Write two mechanism of Na^+ absorption.
12. Enumerate three functions of juxtaglomerular cells.

Abdomen:

Date:

Station no. 24: Palpate the liver of a given subject by classical method and report your findings.

Domains tested: Psychomotor, affective and communication

S. no.	Steps	Marks	R. no. 1	R. no. 2	R. no. 3
A.	**Checklist**				
1.	Stands on the right side of the subject	1			
2.	Explains detail procedure and takes verbal consent	1			
3.	Exposes the abdomen fully up to just above the xiphisternum	1			
4.	Ensures that his own hands are warm	1			
5.	Asks the subject to breath quietly	1			
6.	Places his both hands side by side flat on the abdomen of the subject in the right subcostal region with fingers pointing towards the ribs	4			
7.	Asks the subject to breath in deeply and at the height of the inspiration presses the finger firmly inwards and upwards	2			
8.	Narrates the findings to the observer	1			
9.	Covers the exposed area properly	1			
B.	**Assessment of Professional Behavior**				
1.	Informs subject regarding completion of procedure and thanks the subject	1			
	Total Marks	14			
	Correction Factor				
	Final Score				
	Global Rating: 1. Poor; 2. Unsatisfactory; 3. Satisfactory; 4. Good; 5. Excellent				
Observer's Comment (based on general observation):					
Signature of Observer					

Response stations:

1. List the four functions of liver.
2. Enlist any four gastrointestinal hormones and give one function of each.
3. Enumerate any four functions of gallbladder.
4. Enumerate any four liver function tests.
5. Name any four substances synthesized in liver.
6. Write two causes of hepatomegaly.

Abdomen: Date:

Station no. 25: Palpate the spleen of a given subject by classical method and report your findings.

Domains tested: Psychomotor, affective and communication

S. no.	Steps	Marks	R. no. 1	R. no. 2	R. no. 3
A.	**Checklist**				
1.	Stands on the right side of the subject	1			
2.	Explains detail procedure and takes verbal consent	1			
3.	Exposes the abdomen fully up to just above the xiphisternum	1			
4.	Ensures that his own hands are warm	1			
5.	Asks the subject to breath quietly	1			
6.	Places the flat of the left hand over the lowermost rib cage posterolaterally and the right hand beneath the costal margin in the left hypochondriac region	4			
7.	Asks the subject to breath in deeply, press in deeply with the fingers of the right hand beneath the costal margin at the same time exerting pressure medially and downwards with the left hand	2			
8.	Repeats the procedure with the right hand being moving more medially beneath the costal margin on each occasion	2			
9.	Narrates the findings to the observer	1			
10.	Covers the exposed area properly	1			
B.	**Assessment of Professional Behavior**				
1.	Informs subject regarding completion of procedure and thanks the subject	1			
	Total Marks	**16**			
	Correction Factor				
	Final Score				
	Global Rating: 1. Poor; 2. Unsatisfactory; 3. Satisfactory; 4. Good; 5. Excellent				
	Observer's Comment (based on general observation):				
	Signature of Observer				

Response stations:
1. List two functions of spleen.
2. Enlist any four gastrointestinal hormones and give one function of each.
3. Write two causes of splenomegaly.

Abdomen: Date:

Station no. 26: Elicit fluid thrill in a given subject and report your findings.

Domains tested: Psychomotor, affective and communication

S. no.	Steps	Marks	R. no. 1	R. no. 2	R. no. 3
A.	**Checklist**				
1.	Stands on the right side of the subject	1			
2.	Explains detail procedure and takes verbal consent	1			
3.	Exposes the abdomen fully up to just above the xiphisternum	1			
4.	Places one hand flat over the lumbar region laterally on left side	2			
5.	Gets the assistance to put the side of his hand firmly in the midline of the abdomen	2			
6.	Taps or flicks the opposite side of lumbar region, i.e. from right side	2			
7.	Narrates the findings to the observer	1			
8.	Covers the exposed area properly	1			
B.	**Assessment of Professional Behavior**				
1.	Informs subject regarding completion of procedure and thanks the subject	1			
	Total Marks	**12**			
	Correction Factor				
	Final Score				
	Global Rating: 1. Poor; 2. Unsatisfactory; 3. Satisfactory; 4. Good; 5. Excellent				
Observer's Comment (based on general observation):					
Signature of Observer					

Response stations:

1. Write two causes of ascites.
2. What is an ascitic tap?
3. What are the indications for ascitic tap?
4. Enlist any four gastrointestinal hormones and give one function of each.
5. List the four functions of liver.
6. Enumerate any four liver function tests.
7. Name any four substances synthesized in liver.

Abdomen: Date:

Station no. 27: Percuss for the upper border of liver and report your findings.

Domains tested: Psychomotor, affective and communication

S. no.	Steps	Marks	R. no. 1	R. no. 2	R. no. 3
A.	**Checklist**				
1.	Stands on the right side of the subject	1			
2.	Explains detail procedure and takes verbal consent	1			
3.	Exposes the abdomen fully up to just above the xiphisternum	1			
4.	Locates the 2nd intercostal space on right side	2			
5.	Starts percussing from 2nd intercostal space (resonant note) going downwards till the percussion note becomes dull	4			
6.	Identifies that intercostal space and narrates the findings to the observer	2			
7.	Covers the exposed area properly	1			
B.	**Assessment of Professional Behavior**				
1.	Informs subject regarding completion of procedure and thanks the subject	1			
	Total Marks	**13**			
	Correction Factor				
	Final Score				
	Global Rating: 1. Poor; 2. Unsatisfactory; 3. Satisfactory; 4. Good; 5. Excellent				
Observer's Comment (based on general observation):					
Signature of Observer					

Response stations:
1. List the four functions of liver.
2. Enlist any four gastrointestinal hormones and give one function of each.
3. Enumerate any four functions of gallbladder.
4. Enumerate any four liver function tests.
5. Name any four substances synthesized in liver.
6. Write two causes of hepatomegaly.

Abdomen: Date:

Station no. 28: Perform shifting dullness in a given subject and report your findings.

Domains tested: Psychomotor, affective and communication

S. no.	Steps	Marks	R. no. 1	R. no. 2	R. no. 3
A.	**Checklist**				
1.	Stands on the right side of the subject	1			
2.	Explains detail procedure and takes verbal consent	1			
3.	Exposes the abdomen fully up to just above the xiphisternum	1			
4.	Keeps the pleximeter finger of a hand in centre of the abdomen in longitudinal axis	2			
5.	Starts percussing from midline and going towards laterally till dull note is observed	2			
6.	Keeping the hand in the same position on the abdomen, asks the subject to roll away on the opposite side of the hand	2			
7.	Percusses again in the same position	2			
8.	Repeats the procedure on other side	4			
9.	Narrates the findings to the observer	1			
10.	Covers the exposed area properly	1			
B.	**Assessment of Professional Behavior**				
1.	Informs subject regarding completion of procedure and thanks the subject	1			
	Total Marks	**18**			
	Correction Factor				
	Final Score				
	Global Rating: 1. Poor; 2. Unsatisfactory; 3. Satisfactory; 4. Good; 5. Excellent				
Observer's Comment (based on general observation):					
Signature of Observer					

Response stations:
1. Write two causes of ascites.
2. What is an ascitic tap?
3. What are the indications for ascitic tap?
4. Enlist any four gastrointestinal hormones and give one function of each.
5. List the four functions of liver.
6. Enumerate any four liver function tests.
7. Name any four substances synthesized in liver.

Abdomen: Date:

Station no. 29: Perform horseshoe-shaped dullness in a given subject and report your findings.

Domains tested: Psychomotor, affective and communication

S. no.	Steps	Marks	R. no. 1	R. no. 2	R. no. 3
A.	**Checklist**				
1.	Stands on the right side of the subject	1			
2.	Explains detailed procedure and takes verbal consent	1			
3.	Exposes the abdomen fully up to just above the xiphisternum	1			
4.	Starts percussing from umbilicus towards the flanks in all directions	2			
5.	Marks the position of dull note at every point	2			
6.	Connects all the points	2			
7.	Narrates the findings to the observer	1			
8.	Covers the exposed area properly	1			
B.	**Assessment of Professional Behavior**				
1.	Informs subject regarding completion of procedure and thanks the subject	1			
	Total Marks	**12**			
	Correction Factor				
	Final Score				
	Global Rating: 1. Poor; 2. Unsatisfactory; 3. Satisfactory; 4. Good; 5. Excellent				
Observer's Comment (based on general observation):					
Signature of Observer					

Response stations:
1. Write two causes of ascites.
2. What is an ascitic tap?
3. What are the indications for ascitic tap?
4. Enlist any four gastrointestinal hormones and give one function of each.
5. List the four functions of liver.
6. Enumerate any four liver function tests.
7. Name any four substances synthesized in liver.

Abdomen: Date:

Station no. 30: Auscultate for the abdominal sounds in a given subject and report your findings.

Domains tested: Psychomotor, affective and communication

S. no.	Steps	Marks	R. no. 1	R. no. 2	R. no. 3
A.	**Checklist**				
1.	Stands on the right side of the subject	1			
2.	Explains detailed procedure and takes verbal consent	1			
3.	Exposes the abdomen fully up to just above the xiphisternum	1			
4.	Checks for the normal functioning of the stethoscope	1			
5.	Places the diaphragm of the stethoscope with firm pressure over all four quadrants of abdomen simultaneously	4			
6.	Waits for minimum of 30–60 sec at each quadrant to confirm the presence of abdominal sounds	4			
7.	Narrates the findings to the observer	1			
8.	Covers the exposed area properly.	1			
B.	**Assessment of Professional Behavior**				
1.	Informs subject regarding completion of procedure and thanks the subject	1			
	Total Marks	**15**			
	Correction Factor				
	Final Score				
	Global Rating: 1. Poor; 2. Unsatisfactory; 3. Satisfactory; 4. Good; 5. Excellent				
Observer's Comment (based on general observation):					
Signature of Observer					

Response stations:
1. What are borborygmi sounds?
2. What are the causes of absent abdominal sounds?
3. What are the causes of increased abdominal sounds?

Central Nervous System: Cranial Nerves   Date:

Station no. 31: Examine I cranial nerve of a given subject and report your findings.

Domains tested: Cognitive, psychomotor, affective and communication

S. no.	Steps	Marks	R. no. 1	R. no. 2	R. no. 3
A.	**Checklist**				
1.	Stands on the right side of the subject	1			
2.	Explains the procedure and takes verbal consent for examination	1			
3.	Asks the subject to close both eyes	1			
4.	Takes cotton bud and applies clove oil/peppermint oil on it	2			
5.	Applies the cotton bud on each nostril separately	2			
6.	Asks the subject to identify the smell with eyes closed	2			
7.	Narrates findings to the observer	1			
B.	**Assessment of Professional Behavior**				
1.	Informs subject regarding completion of procedure and thanks the subject	1			
	Total Marks	**12**			
	Correction Factor				
	Final Score				
	Global Rating: 1. Poor; 2. Unsatisfactory; 3. Satisfactory; 4. Good; 5. Excellent				
Observer's Comment (based on general observation):					
Signature of Observer					

Response stations:

1. Draw a diagram of olfactory pathway.
2. Define parosmia and anosmia.

Central Nervous System: Cranial Nerves   Date:

Station no. 32: Examine II cranial nerve of a given subject for color vision and report your findings.

Domains tested: Cognitive, psychomotor, affective and communication

S. no.	Steps	Marks	R. no. 1	R. no. 2	R. no. 3
A.	**Checklist**				
1.	Stands on the right side of the subject	1			
2.	Explains the procedure and takes verbal consent for examination	1			
3.	Asks the subject to hold Ishihara chart at a distance of 75 cm from the subject in natural daylight	2			
4.	Asks the subject to read numbers on Plate I, II, and III within 3 seconds	2			
5.	Asks the subject to trace winding lines in plate IV and V with a brush within 10 sec, if the subject was unable to do step 4	2			
6.	Narrates findings to the observer	1			
B.	**Assessment of Professional Behavior**				
1.	Informs subject regarding completion of procedure and thanks the subject	1			
	Total Marks	**11**			
	Correction Factor				
	Final Score				
	Global Rating: 1. Poor; 2. Unsatisfactory; 3. Satisfactory; 4. Good; 5. Excellent				
Observer's Comment (based on general observation):					
Signature of Observer					

Response stations:
1. Draw a labeled diagram of layers of retina.
2. Draw visual cycle in humans.

Central Nervous System: Cranial Nerves   Date:

Station no. 33a: Examine III, IV, VI cranial nerves of a given subject for movement of eyeball and report your findings.

Domains tested: Cognitive, psychomotor, affective and communication

S. no.	Steps	Marks	R. no. 1	R. no. 2	R. no. 3
A.	**Checklist**				
1.	Stands on the right side of the subject	1			
2.	Explains the procedure and takes verbal consent for examination	1			
3.	Asks the subject to close one eye with ipsilateral hand	1			
4.	Asks the subject to follow the movement of examiner's index finger with the open eyes in superior, medial, inferior, lateral and oblique directions	5			
5.	Repeats the same procedure with the other eye	5			
6.	Narrates findings to the observer	1			
B.	**Assessment of Professional Behavior**				
1.	Informs subject regarding completion of procedure and thanks the subject	1			
	Total Marks	**15**			
	Correction Factor				
	Final Score				
	Global Rating: 1. Poor; 2. Unsatisfactory; 3. Satisfactory; 4. Good; 5. Excellent				
Observer's Comment (based on general observation):					
Signature of Observer					

Central Nervous System: Cranial Nerves   Date:

Station no. 33b: Examine III cranial nerve of a given subject for light reflex and report your findings.

Domains tested: Cognitive, psychomotor, affective and communication

S. no.	Steps	Marks	R. no. 1	R. no. 2	R. no. 3
A.	**Checklist**				
1.	Stands on the right side of the subject	1			
2.	Explains the procedure and takes verbal consent for examination	1			
3.	Asks the subject to sit in front of an indirectly illuminated bright light	1			
4.	Asks the subject to close one eye with ipsilateral hand	1			
5.	Asks the subject to look at a distant object	1			
6.	Shows a bright light into the open eye with a torch	2			
7.	Looks for consensual light reflex by opening the other eye	2			
8.	Switches off the torch light	1			
9.	Repeats the same procedure with the other eye	4			
10.	Narrates findings to the observer	1			
B.	**Assessment of Professional Behavior**				
1.	Informs subject regarding completion of procedure and thanks the subject	1			
	Total Marks	**16**			
	Correction Factor				
	Final Score				
	Global Rating: 1. Poor; 2. Unsatisfactory; 3. Satisfactory; 4. Good; 5. Excellent				
Observer's Comment (based on general observation):					
Signature of Observer					

Response stations:
1. Draw the pathway for light reflex.
2. Define direct and consensual (indirect) light reflex.

Central Nervous System: Cranial Nerves   Date:

Station No. 33c: Examine III cranial nerve of a given subject for accommodation reflex and report your findings.

Domains tested: Cognitive, psychomotor, affective and communication

S. no.	Steps	Marks	R. no. 1	R. no. 2	R. no. 3
A.	**Checklist**				
1.	Stands on the right side of the subject	1			
2.	Explains the procedure and takes verbal consent for examination	1			
3.	Holds examiner's index finger close to subjects nose	1			
4.	Asks the subject to look at a distant object	2			
5.	Asks the subject to suddenly look at examiner's index finger	2			
6.	Narrates findings to the observer regarding contraction of ciliary muscle, constriction of pupil and convergence of visual axes	1			
B.	**Assessment of Professional Behavior**				
1.	Informs subject regarding completion of procedure and thanks the subject	1			
	Total Marks	**9**			
	Correction Factor				
	Final Score				
	Global Rating: 1. Poor; 2. Unsatisfactory; 3. Satisfactory; 4. Good; 5. Excellent				
Observer's Comment (based on general observation):					
Signature of Observer					

Response stations:

1. Enumerate the muscles supplied by the III cranial nerve.

Central Nervous System: Cranial Nerves Date:

Station no. 34: Examine V cranial nerve of a given subject and report your findings.

Domains tested: Cognitive, psychomotor, affective and communication

S. no.	Steps	Marks	R. no. 1	R. no. 2	R. no. 3
A.	**Checklist**				
1.	Stands on the right side of the subject	1			
2.	Explains the procedure and takes verbal consent for examination	1			
3.	Asks the subject to close both eyes	1			
4.	Touches parts of face symmetrically (all 3 divisions) on both sides with a wisp of cotton and asks the subject to identify the sensation and locate the area of sensation, with eyes closed	2			
5.	Repeats the above examination with a hypodermic needle to test for superficial pain sensation	2			
6.	Repeats the above examination with warm and cold water in a test tube	2			
7.	Asks the subject to look at a distant object and then touches the cornea at its conjunctival margin with a cotton swab	2			
8.	Repeats step 7 with the other eye	2			
9.	Narrates findings to the observer regarding touch, pain, thermal sensations of face and corneal reflex of both eyes	2			
B.	**Assessment of Professional Behavior**				
1.	Informs subject regarding completion of procedure and thanks the subject	1			
	Total Marks	**16**			
	Correction Factor				
	Final Score				
	Global Rating: 1. Poor; 2. Unsatisfactory; 3. Satisfactory; 4. Good; 5. Excellent				
Observer's Comment (based on general observation):					
Signature of Observer					

Response stations:

1. Write the functions of trigeminal nerve.

Central Nervous System: Cranial Nerves   Date:

Station no. 35: Examine VII cranial nerve of a given subject and report your findings.

Domains tested: Cognitive, psychomotor, affective and communication

S. no.	Steps	Marks	R. no. 1	R. no. 2	R. no. 3
A.	**Checklist**				
1.	Stands on the right side of the subject	1			
2.	Explains the procedure and takes verbal consent for examination	1			
3.	Asks the subject to smile	2			
4.	Asks the subject to close eyes tightly while the examiner tries to open eyes forcefully	2			
5.	Asks the subject to whistle	2			
6.	Asks the subject to frown his forehead	2			
7.	Narrates findings to the observer regarding symmetry of face, facial expression, angle of mouth and findings of examination stated above	1			
B.	**Assessment of Professional Behavior**				
1.	Informs subject regarding completion of procedure and thanks the subject	1			
	Total Marks	**12**			
	Correction Factor				
	Final Score				
	Global Rating: 1. Poor; 2. Unsatisfactory; 3. Satisfactory; 4. Good; 5. Excellent				
Observer's Comment (based on general observation):					
Signature of Observer					

Response stations:

1. Write the functions of facial nerve.
2. Explain pathophysiology and clinical features of Bell's palsy.

Central Nervous System: Cranial Nerves   Date:

Station no. 36: Perform Rinne's test in a given subject and report your findings.

Domains tested: Cognitive, psychomotor, affective and communication

S. no.	Steps	Marks	R. no. 1	R. no. 2	R. no. 3
A.	**Checklist**				
1.	Stands on the right side of the subject	1			
2.	Explains the procedure and takes verbal consent for examination	1			
3.	Asks the subject to close external auditory meatus of opposite ear	2			
4.	Vibrates the tuning fork (256/516 Hz) and keeps its base on the mastoid process of the test ear	2			
5.	Transfers the base of tuning fork close to the ear as soon as the subject ceased hearing the vibrations from mastoid process	2			
6.	Repeats the examination for the other ear	6			
7.	Narrates findings to the observer	1			
B.	**Assessment of Professional Behavior**				
1.	Informs subject regarding completion of procedure and thanks the subject	1			
	Total Marks	**16**			
	Correction Factor				
	Final Score				
	Global Rating: 1. Poor; 2. Unsatisfactory; 3. Satisfactory; 4. Good; 5. Excellent				
Observer's Comment (based on general observation):					
Signature of Observer					

Response stations:

1. Define conductive and neural deafness.
2. How will you identify conductive deafness based on Rinne's test?

Central Nervous System: Cranial Nerves   Date:

Station no. 37: Examine X cranial nerve in a given subject and report your findings.

Domains tested: Cognitive, psychomotor, affective and communication

S. no.	Steps	Marks	R. no. 1	R. no. 2	R. no. 3
A.	**Checklist**				
1.	Stands on the right side of the subject	1			
2.	Explains the procedure and takes verbal consent for examination	1			
3.	Asks the subject about any history of regurgitation of fluids through nose during swallowing	2			
4.	Asks the subject to open mouth widely and say "Ah" and observes the movement of palatal arch	2			
5.	Narrates findings to the observer	2			
B.	**Assessment of Professional Behavior**				
1.	Informs subject regarding completion of procedure and thanks the subject	1			
	Total Marks	**9**			
	Correction Factor				
	Final Score				
	Global Rating: 1. Poor; 2. Unsatisfactory; 3. Satisfactory; 4. Good; 5. Excellent				
Observer's Comment (based on general observation):					
Signature of Observer					

Response stations:

1. Enumerate the divisions and functions of X cranial nerve.

Central Nervous System: Cranial Nerves   Date:

Station no. 38a: Examine XI cranial nerve in a given subject and report your findings.
Domains tested: Cognitive, psychomotor, affective and communication

S. no.	Steps	Marks	R. no. 1	R. no. 2	R. no. 3
A.	**Checklist**				
1.	Stands on the right side of the subject	1			
2.	Explains the procedure and takes verbal consent for examination	2			
3.	Asks the subject to flex his head against resistance	2			
4.	Applies passive resistance from opposite side while the subject rotated his chin to one side	2			
5.	Asks the subject to shrug his shoulders while the examiner applies passive resistance from above	2			
6.	Narrates findings to the observer	2			
B.	**Assessment of Professional Behavior**				
1.	Informs subject regarding completion of procedure and thanks the subject	1			
	Total Marks	**12**			
	Correction Factor				
	Final Score				
	Global Rating: 1. Poor; 2. Unsatisfactory; 3. Satisfactory; 4. Good; 5. Excellent				
Observer's Comment (based on general observation):					
Signature of Observer					

Response stations:
1. Enumerate the muscles supplied by XI cranial nerve.

Central Nervous System: Cranial Nerves   Date:

Station no. 38b: Examine XII cranial nerve in a given subject and report your findings.

Domains tested: Cognitive, psychomotor, affective and communication

S. no.	Steps	Marks	R. no. 1	R. no. 2	R. no. 3
A.	Checklist				
1.	Stands on the right side of the subject	1			
2.	Explains the procedure and takes verbal consent for examination	2			
3.	Asks the subject to open his mouth and inspects the tongue for atrophy/wasting or fasciculations	2			
4.	Asks the subject to protrude the tongue and move from side-to-side	2			
5.	Asks the subjects to stick the tongue out against inside of the cheeks and applies passive resistance with his/her fingers or palm	2			
6.	Narrates findings to the observer	2			
B.	Assessment of Professional Behavior				
1.	Informs subject regarding completion of procedure and thanks the subject	1			
	Total Marks	12			
	Correction Factor				
	Final Score				
	Global Rating: 1. Poor; 2. Unsatisfactory; 3. Satisfactory; 4. Good; 5. Excellent				
Observer's Comment (based on general observation):					
Signature of Observer					

Response stations:

1. Enumerate the muscles supplied by XII cranial nerve.

Central Nervous System: Cranial Nerves　　　　　　　Date:

Station no. 39: Perform confrontation test in a given subject and report your findings.

Domains tested: Cognitive, psychomotor, affective and communication

S. no.	Steps	Marks	R. no. 1	R. no. 2	R. no. 3
A.	**Checklist**				
1.	Stands on the right side of the subject	1			
2.	Explains the procedure and takes verbal consent for examination	1			
3.	The examiner sits in front of the subject at a distance of half meter	1			
4.	Examiner and subject, while sitting opposite to each other; closes one eye of same side with their hand	2			
5.	Holds his hand (examiners') with index finger raised, on the side of open eye of subject, at full arm's length and slowly brings it in front of the open eye of the subject	2			
6.	Asks the subject to indicate when he stops visualizing the index finger while bringing it near to the open eye and while regaining the visual	1			
7.	Performs step 6 in all 4 quadrants—upwards, downwards, right and left	4			
8.	Repeats step 4–7 for the other eye	4			
9.	Narrates findings to the observer	1			
B.	**Assessment of Professional Behavior**				
1.	Informs subject regarding completion of procedure and thanks the subject	1			
	Total Marks	**18**			
	Correction Factor				
	Final Score				
	Global Rating: 1. Poor; 2. Unsatisfactory; 3. Satisfactory; 4. Good; 5. Excellent				
Observer's Comment (based on general observation):					
Signature of Observer					

Response stations:

1. Apart from confrontation test, identify other methods by which one can assess field of vision.

Central Nervous System: Motor System   Date:

Station no. 40: Examine for power of muscle in upper extremity of a given subject and report your findings.

Domains tested: Cognitive, psychomotor, affective and communication

S. no.	Steps	Marks	R. no. 1	R. no. 2	R. no. 3
A.	**Checklist**				
1.	Stands on the right side of the subject	1			
2.	Explains the procedure and takes verbal consent for examination	1			
3.	Asks the subject to flex metacarpophalangeal joint and extend distal interphalangeal joint	2			
4.	Asks the subject to squeeze examiner's fingers	2			
5.	Asks the subject to bring tips of his fingers towards front of his forearm	2			
6.	Asks the subject to flex his wrist	2			
7.	Asks the subject to place forearm in mid-prone position and then flex it against resistance	2			
8.	Asks the subject to place forearm in full supination and then flex against resistance	2			
9.	Asks the subject to place forearm fully flexed against the chest and then asks to straighten it (extend) against resistance	2			
10.	Asks the subject to lift his arm at right angles to his side against resistance	2			
11.	Repeats the steps 3–10 on opposite side of upper extremity	16			
12.	Narrates findings to the observer with regards to muscles of upper extremity	1			
B.	**Assessment of Professional Behavior**				
1.	Informs subject regarding completion of procedure and thanks the subject	1			
	Total Marks	**36**			
	Correction Factor				
	Final Score				
	Global Rating: 1. Poor; 2. Unsatisfactory; 3. Satisfactory; 4. Good; 5. Excellent				
Observer's Comment (based on general observation):					
Signature of Observer					

Response stations:
1. State the grading of power of muscles.
2. Identify any two conditions wherein muscle power is decreased.

Central Nervous System: Motor System   Date:

Station no. 41: Examine for power of muscle in lower extremity of a given subject and report your findings.

Domains tested: Cognitive, psychomotor, affective and communication

S. no.	Steps	Marks	R. no. 1	R. no. 2	R. no. 3
A.	**Checklist**				
1.	Stands on the right side of the subject	1			
2.	Explains the procedure and takes verbal consent for examination	1			
3.	Asks the subject to elevate and depress the toes against resistance	2			
4.	Asks the subject to flex his knee and then straighten it against resistance	2			
5.	Gives supine position to the subject, raises his leg from the bed supporting thigh with one hand and ankle with other hand and then asks the subject to flex his legs	2			
6.	Repeats the steps 3–5 on opposite side of upper extremity	2			
7.	Narrates findings to the observer with regards to muscles of upper extremity	2			
B.	**Assessment of Professional Behavior**				
1.	Informs subject regarding completion of procedure and thanks the subject	1			
	Total Marks	**13**			
	Correction Factor				
	Final Score				
	Global Rating: 1. Poor; 2. Unsatisfactory; 3. Satisfactory; 4. Good; 5. Excellent				
Observer's Comment (based on general observation):					
Signature of Observer					

Response stations:

1. State the grading of power of muscles.
2. Identify any two conditions wherein muscle power is decreased.

Central Nervous System: Motor System   Date:

Station no. 42: Examine for co-ordination in upper limb of a given subject and report your findings.

Domains tested: Cognitive, psychomotor, affective and communication

S. no.	Steps	Marks	R. no. 1	R. no. 2	R. no. 3
A.	**Checklist**				
1.	Stands on the right side of the subject	1			
2.	Explains the procedure and takes verbal consent for examination	1			
3.	Asks the subject to first touch his nose with index finger and then examiner's index finger with eyes open for 5–6 times	2			
4.	Asks the subject to first touch his nose with index finger and then examiner's index finger with closed eyes for 5–6 times	2			
5.	Asks the subject to draw circle in air with index finger, first with eyes closed and then with eyes open	2			
6.	Asks the subject to do rapid pronation and supination of the forearm	2			
7.	Narrates findings to the observer with regards to muscles of upper extremity	2			
B.	**Assessment of Professional Behavior**				
1.	Informs subject regarding completion of procedure and thanks the subject	1			
	Total Marks	**13**			
	Correction Factor				
	Final Score				
	Global Rating: 1. Poor; 2. Unsatisfactory; 3. Satisfactory; 4. Good; 5. Excellent				
Observer's Comment (based on general observation):					
Signature of Observer					

Response stations:
1. State the sensation carried by dorsal column tract.
2. State the sensation carried by lateral spinothalamic tract.
3. State the sensation carried by anterior spinothalamic tract.

Central Nervous System: Motor System Date:

Station No. 43: Examine for co-ordination in lower limb of a given subject and report your findings.

Domains tested: Cognitive, psychomotor, affective and communication

S. no.	Steps	Marks	R. no. 1	R. no. 2	R. no. 3
A.	**Checklist**				
1.	Stands on the right side of the subject	1			
2.	Explains the procedure and takes verbal consent for examination	1			
3.	Asks the subject to walk along in straight line with eyes open	2			
4.	Asks the subject to walk along in straight line with eyes closed	2			
5.	Asks the subject to place the heel of one leg over the knee and then slide over the shin of tibia towards the ankle	2			
6.	Narrates findings to the observer with regards to muscles of upper extremity	2			
B.	**Assessment of Professional Behavior**				
1.	Informs subject regarding completion of procedure and thanks the subject	1			
	Total Marks	**11**			
	Correction Factor				
	Final Score				
	Global Rating: 1. Poor; 2. Unsatisfactory; 3. Satisfactory; 4. Good; 5. Excellent				
Observer's Comment (based on general observation):					
Signature of Observer					

Response stations:
1. Define dysdiadochokinesia
2. Define cerebellar and motor ataxia.

Central Nervous System: Motor System   Date:

Station no. 44: Assess the tone of flexors for upper limb elbow joint of a given subject and report your findings.

Domains tested: Cognitive, psychomotor, affective and communication

S. no.	Steps	Marks	R. no. 1	R. no. 2	R. no. 3
A.	**Checklist**				
1.	Stands on the right side of the subject	1			
2.	Explains the procedure and takes verbal consent for examination	1			
3.	Makes passive flexion and extension movements at the elbow joint	2			
4.	Feels the tone of flexors and extensors	2			
5.	Compares the findings with the opposite side	2			
6.	Narrates findings to the observer	2			
B.	**Assessment of Professional Behavior**				
1.	Informs subject regarding completion of procedure and thanks the subject	1			
	Total Marks	**11**			
	Correction Factor				
	Final Score				
	Global Rating: 1. Poor; 2. Unsatisfactory; 3. Satisfactory; 4. Good; 5. Excellent				
Observer's Comment (based on general observation):					
Signature of Observer					

Response stations:
1. Define muscle tone.
2. Write causes of hypotonia.
3. Write causes of hypertonia.

Central Nervous System: Motor System   Date:

Station no. 45: Assess the tone of a muscle in lower limb knee joint of a given subject and report your findings.

Domains tested: Cognitive, psychomotor, affective and communication

S. no.	Steps	Marks	R. no. 1	R. no. 2	R. no. 3
A.	**Checklist**				
1.	Stands on the right side of the subject	1			
2.	Explains the procedure and takes verbal consent for examination	1			
3.	Makes passive flexion and extension movements at the knee joint	2			
4.	Feels the tone of flexors and extensors	2			
5.	Compares the findings with the opposite side	2			
6.	Narrates findings to the observer	2			
B.	**Assessment of Professional Behavior**				
1.	Informs subject regarding completion of procedure and thanks the subject	1			
	Total Marks	**11**			
	Correction Factor				
	Final Score				
	Global Rating: 1. Poor; 2. Unsatisfactory; 3. Satisfactory; 4. Good; 5. Excellent				
Observer's Comment (based on general observation):					
Signature of Observer					

Response stations:
1. Define tone.
2. Explain in short, the basis of muscle tone.

Central Nervous System: Reflexes   Date:

Station no. 46: Elicit biceps jerk in a given subject in sitting position and report your findings.

Domains tested: Cognitive, psychomotor, affective and communication

S. no.	Steps	Marks	R. no. 1	R. no. 2	R. no. 3
A.	**Checklist**				
1.	Takes proper consent to perform the procedure	1			
2.	Orients the patient about the procedure in local language	1			
3.	Asks the subject to expose the part to be examined	0.5			
4.	Asks the subject to relax	1			
5.	Flexes the subject's elbow to right angle and places forearm of the subject in semi-pronated position supported by examiner's hand	1.5			
6.	Makes the subject to rest his forearm on the forearm of the examiner	1			
7.	Locates the tendon of biceps	1			
8.	Places own thumb on the bicep's tendon	1			
9.	Strikes own thumb with the pointed end of the knee hammer	2			
10.	Compares with the biceps jerk on the opposite side	1			
11.	Narrates the findings to the observer regarding: Contraction of the biceps muscle Flexion at the elbow joint Level of spinal cord involved	3			
B.	**Assessment of Professional Behavior**				
1.	Informs subject regarding completion of procedure and thanks the subject	1			
	Total Marks	**15**			
	Correction Factor				
	Final Score				
	Global Rating: 1. Poor; 2. Unsatisfactory; 3. Satisfactory; 4. Good; 5. Excellent				
Observer's Comment (based on general observation):					
Signature of Observer					

Response stations:
1. Differentiate between superficial and deep reflexes.
2. Enumerate the four superficial reflexes.
3. Enumerate the four deep reflexes.

4. Describe adequate stimulus.
5. Enumerate the four components of reflex arc.
6. Enumerate the components of a stretch reflex.
7. Enumerate properties of reflexes.
8. Enumerate four cutaneous receptors
9. Enumerate the components of inverse stretch reflex
10. A 33-yr-old male was admitted through the emergency room with neck pain, and loss of sensation and inability to move all four extremities. He had crashed his car into the post of a traffic signal, was not wearing a seat belt, and the front air bag deployed. On neurologic examination, the patient had flaccid paralysis of all four extremities.

    What will be elicited on the examination of deep reflexes in the patient?
11. A male patient aged 60 years, reported early in morning in OPD with complain of loss of movements and weakness of the right half side of the body.
    a. What shall be diagnosis of the patient and what will be your observation on clinical examination of plantar reflex on the affected side?
12. A female patient of 60 years of age had suddenly developed the weakness of left side of the body with complains of excruciating pain. On clinical examination, muscle tone was decreased on affected side with loss of power of muscles and plantar reflex showing Babinski's positive.

    What is the site of lesion in this patient?

Central Nervous System: Reflexes   Date:

Station no. 47: Elicit biceps jerk in a given subject in supine position and report your findings.

Domains tested: Cognitive, psychomotor, affective and communication

S. no.	Steps	Marks	R. no. 1	R. no. 2	R. no. 3
A.	**Checklist**				
1.	Takes proper consent to perform the procedure	1			
2.	Orients the patient about the procedure in local language	1			
3.	Asks the subject to expose the part to be examined	0.5			
4.	Asks the subject to relax	1			
5.	Flexes the subject's elbow to right angle and places forearm of the subject in semi-pronated position supported by examiner's hand	1.5			
6.	Makes the subject to rest his forearm on the forearm of the examiner	1			
7.	Locates the tendon of biceps	1			
8.	Places own thumb on the bicep's tendon	1			
9.	Strikes own thumb with the pointed end of the knee hammer	2			
10.	Compares with the biceps jerk on the opposite side	1			
11.	Narrates the findings to the observer regarding: Contraction of the biceps muscle Flexion at the elbow joint Level of spinal cord involved	3			
B.	**Assessment of Professional Behavior**				
1.	Informs subject regarding completion of procedure and thanks the subject	1			
	Total Marks	**15**			
	Correction Factor				
	Final Score				
	Global Rating: 1. Poor; 2. Unsatisfactory; 3. Satisfactory; 4. Good; 5. Excellent				
Observer's Comment (based on general observation):					
Signature of Observer					

Central Nervous System: Reflexes Date:

Station no. 48a: Elicit triceps jerk in a given subject in sitting position and report your findings.

Domains tested: Cognitive, psychomotor, affective and communication

S. no.	Steps	Marks	R. no. 1	R. no. 2	R. no. 3
A.	**Checklist**				
1.	Takes proper consent to perform the procedure	1			
2.	Orients the patient about the procedure in local language	1			
3.	Asks the subject to expose the part to be examined	1			
4.	Asks the subject to relax	1			
5.	Flexes the subject's elbow to right angle	1.5			
6.	Makes the subject to rest his forearm on the forearm of the examiner	1.5			
7.	Strikes the triceps tendon by the broad end of the knee hammer directly above the olecranon	2			
8.	Compares with the triceps jerk on the opposite side	1			
9.	Narrates the findings to the observer regarding: Contraction of the triceps muscle Extension at the elbow joint Level of spinal cord involved	3			
B.	**Assessment of Professional Behavior**				
1.	Informs subject regarding completion of procedure and thanks the subject	1			
	Total Marks	**14**			
	Correction Factor				
	Final Score				
	Global Rating: 1. Poor; 2. Unsatisfactory; 3. Satisfactory; 4. Good; 5. Excellent				
Observer's Comment (based on general observation):					
Signature of Observer					

Central Nervous System: Reflexes Date:

Station no. 48b: Elicit triceps jerk in a given subject in supine position and report your findings.

Domains tested: Cognitive, psychomotor, affective and communication

S. no.	Steps	Marks	R. no. 1	R. no. 2	R. no. 3
A.	**Checklist**				
1.	Takes proper consent to perform the procedure	1			
2.	Orients the patient about the procedure in local language	1			
3.	Asks the subject to expose the part to be examined	1			
4.	Asks the subject to relax	1			
5.	Flexes the subject's elbow to right angle	1.5			
6.	Makes the subject to rest his forearm on his abdomen in supine position	1.5			
7.	Strikes the triceps tendon by the broad end of the knee hammer directly above the olecranon	2			
8.	Compares with the triceps jerk on the opposite side	1			
9.	Narrates the findings to the observer regarding: Contraction of the triceps muscle Extension at the elbow joint Level of spinal cord involved	3			
B.	**Assessment of Professional Behavior**				
1.	Informs subject regarding completion of procedure and thanks the subject	1			
	Total Marks	**14**			
	Correction Factor				
	Final Score				
	Global Rating: 1. Poor; 2. Unsatisfactory; 3. Satisfactory; 4. Good; 5. Excellent				
Observer's Comment (based on general observation):					
Signature of Observer					

Central Nervous System: Reflexes Date:

Station no. 49a: Elicit knee jerk in a given subject in sitting position and report your findings.

Domains tested: Psychomotor, affective and communication

S. No.	Steps	Marks	R. No. 1	R. No. 2	R. No. 3
A.	Checklist				
1.	Takes proper consent to perform the procedure	1			
2.	Orients the patient about the procedure in local language	1			
3.	Asks the subject to sit over the edge of the bed with his legs dangling freely down	1			
4.	Asks the subject to expose the part to be examined up to the upper thigh	1			
5.	Asks the subject to relax	1			
6.	Feels for the patellar tendon	2			
7.	Strikes the patellar tendon midway between the origin and insertion with the pointed end of the knee hammer	2			
8.	Compares with the triceps jerk on the opposite side	1			
9.	Narrates the findings to the observer regarding: Contraction of the quadriceps muscle Extension at the knee joint Level of spinal cord involved	3			
B.	Assessment of Professional Behavior				
1.	Informs subject regarding completion of procedure and thanks the subject	1			
	Total Marks	14			
	Correction Factor				
	Final Score				
	Global Rating: 1. Poor; 2. Unsatisfactory; 3. Satisfactory; 4. Good; 5. Excellent				
Observer's Comment (based on general observation):					
Signature of Observer					

Central Nervous System: Reflexes   Date:

Station no. 49b: Elicit knee jerk in a given subject in supine position and report your findings.

Domains tested: Cognitive, psychomotor, affective and communication

S. no.	Steps	Marks	R. no. 1	R. no. 2	R. no. 3
A.	**Checklist**				
1.	Takes proper consent to perform the procedure	1			
2.	Orients the patient about the procedure in local language	1			
3.	Asks the subject to semiflex the knee in the supine position	1			
4.	Passes the hand of the examiner under the semi-flexed knee joint of the subject and places the hand on the opposite knee joint	2			
5.	Makes the test knee rest on the dorsum of the examiner's wrist joint	1			
6.	Lifts own hand slightly so as to rest the weight of the knee on the examiner's hand	1			
7.	Strikes the patellar tendon midway between the origin and insertion with the pointed end of the knee hammer	2			
8.	Compares with the knee jerk on the opposite side	1			
9.	Narrates the findings to the observer regarding: Contraction of the quadriceps muscle Extension at the knee joint Level of spinal cord involved	3			
B.	**Assessment of Professional Behavior**				
1.	Informs subject regarding completion of procedure and thanks the subject	1			
	Total Marks	**14**			
	Correction Factor				
	Final Score				
	Global Rating: 1. Poor; 2. Unsatisfactory; 3. Satisfactory; 4. Good; 5. Excellent				
	Observer's Comment (based on general observation):				
	Signature of Observer				

Central Nervous System: Reflexes   Date:

Station no. 50a: Elicit ankle jerk in a given subject in sitting position and report your findings.

Domains tested: Cognitive, psychomotor, affective and communication

S. no.	Steps	Marks	R. no. 1	R. no. 2	R. no. 3
A.	**Checklist**				
1.	Takes proper consent to perform the procedure	1			
2.	Orients the patient about the procedure in local language	1			
3.	Asks the subject to kneel on the chair with legs projecting out from the chair	1			
4.	Asks the subject to expose the lower limb up to the knee joint	1			
5.	Gently holds the foot and dorsiflexes it	1			
6.	Strikes the Achilles tendon with the broad end of the knee hammer	2			
7.	Compares with the knee jerk on the opposite side	1			
8.	Narrates the findings to the observer regarding: Contraction of calf muscles Plantar flexion of the foot Level of spinal cord involved	3			
B.	**Assessment of Professional Behavior**				
1.	Informs subject regarding completion of procedure and thanks the subject	1			
	Total Marks	**12**			
	Correction Factor				
	Final Score				
	Global Rating: 1. Poor; 2. Unsatisfactory; 3. Satisfactory; 4. Good; 5. Excellent				
Observer's Comment (based on general observation):					
Signature of Observer					

Central Nervous System: Reflexes Date:

Station no. 50b: Elicit ankle jerk in a given subject in supine position and report your findings.

Domains tested: Cognitive, psychomotor, affective and communication

S. No.	Steps	Marks	R. No. 1	R. No. 2	R. No. 3
A.	**Checklist**				
1.	Takes proper consent to perform the procedure	1			
2.	Orients the patient about the procedure in local language	1			
3.	Asks the subject to lie in supine position such that his lower limb is everted and slightly flexed	1			
4.	Asks the subject to expose the lower limb up to the knee joint	1			
5.	Gently holds the foot and dorsiflexes it	1			
6.	Strikes the Achilles tendon with the broad end of the knee hammer	2			
7.	Compares with the knee jerk on the opposite side	1			
8.	Narrates the findings to the observer regarding: Contraction of calf muscles Plantar flexion of the foot Level of spinal cord involved	3			
B.	**Assessment of Professional Behavior**				
1.	Informs subject regarding completion of procedure and thanks the subject	1			
	Total Marks	**12**			
	Correction Factor				
	Final Score				
	Global Rating: 1. Poor; 2. Unsatisfactory; 3. Satisfactory; 4. Good; 5. Excellent				
Observer's Comment (based on general observation):					
Signature of Observer					

Central Nervous System: Reflexes Date:

Station no. 51: Elicit plantar reflex in a given subject and report your findings.

Domains tested: Cognitive, psychomotor, affective and communication

S. no.	Steps	Marks	R. no. 1	R. no. 2	R. no. 3
A.	**Checklist**				
1.	Takes proper consent to perform the procedure	1			
2.	Orients the patient about the procedure in local language	1			
3.	Asks the subject to relax the muscle of lower limb in supine position	1			
4.	Grasps the leg just above the ankle joint with one hand	1			
5.	Gently scratches the outer edge of the sole of the foot from the heel towards little toe and then medially across the metatarsals towards great toe with pointed metallic part of knee hammer or pointed key	2			
6.	Compares with the plantar reflex on the opposite side	1			
7.	Narrates the findings to the observer regarding: Inversion and dorsiflexion of the ankle Plantar flexion of all the toes at the metatarsus Level of spinal cord involved	3			
B.	**Assessment of Professional Behavior**				
1.	Informs subject regarding completion of procedure and thanks the subject	1			
	Total Marks	**11**			
	Correction Factor				
	Final Score				
	Global Rating: 1. Poor; 2. Unsatisfactory; 3. Satisfactory; 4. Good; 5. Excellent				
Observer's Comment (based on general observation):					
Signature of Observer					

Central Nervous System: Reflexes   Date:

Station no. 52: Elicit abdominal reflex in a given subject and report your findings.

Domains tested: Cognitive, psychomotor, affective and communication

S. no.	Steps	Marks	R. no. 1	R. no. 2	R. no. 3
A.	**Checklist**				
1.	Takes proper consent to perform the procedure	1			
2.	Orients the patient about the procedure in local language	1			
3.	Asks the subject to lie in supine position	1			
4.	Asks the subject to expose the abdomen	1			
5.	Asks the subject to relax completely	1			
6.	Strokes briskly but lightly with a key from outer aspect towards the midline above and below the umbilicus	2			
7.	Narrates the findings to the observer regarding: Contraction of abdominal muscles Level of spinal cord involved	2			
B.	**Assessment of Professional Behavior**				
1.	Informs subject regarding completion of procedure and thanks the subject	1			
	Total Marks	**10**			
	Correction Factor				
	Final Score				
	Global Rating: 1. Poor; 2. Unsatisfactory; 3. Satisfactory; 4. Good; 5. Excellent				
Observer's Comment (based on general observation):					
Signature of Observer					

Central Nervous System: Reflexes   Date:
Station no. 53: Elicit supinator jerk in a given subject and report your findings.
Domains tested: Cognitive, psychomotor, affective and communication

S. no.	Steps	Marks	R. no. 1	R. no. 2	R. no. 3
A.	**Checklist**				
1.	Takes proper consent to perform the procedure	1			
2.	Orients the patient about the procedure in local language	1			
3.	Places the arm of the subject at right angle	1			
4.	Holds the subject's hand in sitting position	1			
5.	Bends the hand laterally in opposite direction to stretch the brachioradialis muscle	1			
6.	Strokes the radius with pointed end of the knee hammer over its styloid process 1–2 inches above the wrist	2			
7.	Compares with the supinator jerk on the opposite side	1			
8.	Narrates the findings to the observer regarding: Flexion at the elbow Supination of the forearm Level of spinal cord involved	3			
B.	**Assessment of Professional Behavior**				
1.	Informs subject regarding completion of procedure and thanks the subject	1			
	Total Marks	**12**			
	Correction Factor				
	Final Score				
	Global Rating: 1. Poor; 2. Unsatisfactory; 3. Satisfactory; 4. Good; 5. Excellent				
Observer's Comment (based on general observation):					
Signature of Observer					

Central Nervous System: Reflexes   Date:

Station no. 54: Elicit jaw jerk in a given subject and report your findings.

Domains tested: Cognitive, psychomotor, affective and communication

S. no.	Steps	Marks	R. no. 1	R. no. 2	R. no. 3
A.	**Checklist**				
1.	Takes proper consent to perform the procedure	1			
2.	Orients the patient about the procedure in local language	1			
3.	Asks the subject to open mouth partially	1			
4.	Places own finger on chin of the subject	1			
5.	Strikes own finger with the help of narrow end of the knee hammer	2			
6.	Narrates the findings to the observer regarding: Closure of the mouth	1			
B.	**Assessment of Professional Behavior**				
1.	Informs subject regarding completion of procedure and thanks the subject	1			
	Total Marks	**8**			
	Correction Factor				
	Final Score				
	Global Rating: 1. Poor; 2. Unsatisfactory; 3. Satisfactory; 4. Good; 5. Excellent				
Observer's Comment (based on general observation):					
Signature of Observer					

Central Nervous System: Sensory System   Date:

Station no. 55: Examine the given subject for fine touch on forearm anterior aspect and report your findings.

Domains tested: Cognitive, psychomotor, affective and communication

S. no.	Steps	Marks	R. no. 1	R. no. 2	R. no. 3
A.	**Checklist**				
1.	Takes proper consent to perform the procedure	1			
2.	Orients the patient about the procedure in local language	1			
3.	Instructs the subject to say "yes" or lift the opposite hand when he feels fine touch sensation	2			
4.	Asks the subject to close his eyes	2			
5.	Lightly touches the skin with Von Frey's hair aesthesiometer in any dermatome on anterior aspect of forearm	2			
6.	Compares with the same dermatome on the opposite side of the forearm	2			
7.	Narrates the findings to the observer	1			
B.	**Assessment of Professional Behavior**				
1.	Informs subject regarding completion of procedure and thanks the subject	1			
	Total Marks	**12**			
	Correction Factor				
	Final Score				
	Global Rating: 1. Poor; 2. Unsatisfactory; 3. Satisfactory; 4. Good; 5. Excellent				
Observer's Comment (based on general observation):					
Signature of Observer					

Response stations:
1. Enumerate various sensations.
2. Enumerate various tactile receptors.
3. Which tract carries sensation of touch.
4. Draw diagram of tract carrying this sensation.

Central Nervous System: Sensory System   Date:

Station no. 56: Examine the given subject for tactile localization on forearm anterior aspect and report your findings.

Domains tested: Cognitive, psychomotor, affective and communication

S. no.	Steps	Marks	R. no. 1	R. no. 2	R. no. 3
A.	**Checklist**				
1.	Takes proper consent to perform the procedure	1			
2.	Orients the patient about the procedure in local language	1			
3.	Asks the subject to close his eyes	2			
4.	Lightly touches the skin in any dermatome on anterior aspect of forearm with a sketch pen	1.5			
5.	Asks the subject to touch the same point with another sketch pen	1.5			
6.	Compares with the same dermatome on the opposite side of the forearm	2			
7.	Narrates the findings to the observer	1			
B.	**Assessment of Professional Behavior**				
1.	Informs subject regarding completion of procedure and thanks the subject	1			
	Total Marks	**11**			
	Correction Factor				
	Final Score				
	Global Rating: 1. Poor; 2. Unsatisfactory; 3. Satisfactory; 4. Good; 5. Excellent				
	Observer's Comment (based on general observation):				
	Signature of Observer				

Response stations:

1. Enumerate various sensations.
2. Enumerate various tactile receptors.
3. Which tract carries sensation of tactile localization.
4. Draw diagram of tract carrying this sensation.

Central Nervous System: Sensory System   Date:

Station no. 57: Examine the given subject for sensation of pressure on forearm anterior aspect and report your findings.

Domains tested: Cognitive, Psychomotor, Affective and Communication

S. no.	Steps	Marks	R. no. 1	R. no. 2	R. no. 3
A.	**Checklist**				
1.	Takes proper consent to perform the procedure	1			
2.	Orients the patient about the procedure in local language	1			
3.	Asks the subject to close his eyes	2			
4.	Uses any blunt object to elicit pressure sensation on dermatome on anterior aspect of forearm	1.5			
5.	Asks the subject to tell 'yes' every time he feels the sensation	1.5			
6.	Compares with the same dermatome on the opposite side of the forearm	2			
7.	Narrates the findings to the observer	1			
B.	**Assessment of Professional Behavior**				
1.	Informs subject regarding completion of procedure and thanks the subject	1			
	Total Marks	**11**			
	Correction Factor				
	Final Score				
	Global Rating: 1. Poor; 2. Unsatisfactory; 3. Satisfactory; 4. Good; 5. Excellent				
Observer's Comment (based on general observation):					
Signature of Observer					

Response stations:
1. Enumerate various sensations.
2. Enumerate various tactile receptors.
3. Which tract carries sensation of pressure.
4. Draw diagram of tract carrying this sensation.

Central Nervous System: Sensory System   Date:

Station no. 58: Examine the given subject for two-point discrimination on forearm anterior aspect and report your findings.

Domains tested: Cognitive, Psychomotor, Affective and Communication

S. no.	Steps	Marks	R. no. 1	R. no. 2	R. no. 3
A.	**Checklist**				
1.	Takes proper consent to perform the procedure	1			
2.	Orients the patient about the procedure in local language	1			
3.	Asks the subject to close his eyes	2			
4.	Instructs the subject to say whether he perceives sensation of one point or two points when touched by an instrument	1.5			
5.	Touches the skin of a dermatome with the two limbs of compass aesthesiometer slightly separate from each other	1.5			
6.	Asks whether the subject feels as one point or two points	1			
7.	Increases the distance between two points till two separate points are perceived by the subject	1			
8.	Compares with the same dermatome on the opposite side of the forearm	1			
9.	Narrates the findings to the observer inclusive of the minimum separable distance	1			
B.	**Assessment of Professional Behavior**				
1.	Informs subject regarding completion of procedure and thanks the subject	1			
	Total Marks	**12**			
	Correction Factor				
	Final Score				
	Global Rating: 1. Poor; 2. Unsatisfactory; 3. Satisfactory; 4. Good; 5. Excellent				
Observer's Comment (based on general observation):					
Signature of Observer					

Response stations:
1. Enumerate various sensations.
2. Enumerate various tactile receptors.
3. Which tract carries sensation of two-point discrimination.
4. Draw diagram of tract carrying this sensation.

Central Nervous System: Sensory System   Date:

Station no. 59: Examine the given subject for sense of temperature on forearm anterior aspect and report your findings.

Domains tested: Cognitive, psychomotor, affective and communication

S. no.	Steps	Marks	R. no. 1	R. no. 2	R. no. 3
A.	**Checklist**				
1.	Takes proper consent to perform the procedure	1			
2.	Orients the patient about the procedure in local language	1			
3.	Asks the subject to close his eyes	2			
4.	Touches warm water/cold water or warm end / cold end of the thermo-asthesiometer to any dermatome on anterior aspect of forearm randomly	2			
5.	Asks the subject to tell 'warm' or 'cold' every time he feels the sensation	1			
6.	Compares with the same dermatome on the opposite side of the forearm	2			
7.	Narrates the findings to the observer	1			
B.	**Assessment of Professional Behavior**				
1.	Informs subject regarding completion of procedure and thanks the subject	1			
	Total Marks	**11**			
	Correction Factor				
	Final Score				
	Global Rating: 1. Poor; 2. Unsatisfactory; 3. Satisfactory; 4. Good; 5. Excellent				
	Observer's Comment (based on general observation):				
	Signature of Observer				

Response stations:
1. Enumerate various sensations.
2. Enumerate various tactile receptors.
3. Which tract carries sensation of temperature.
4. Draw diagram of tract carrying this sensation.

Central Nervous System: Sensory System   Date:

Station no. 60: Examine the given subject for sense of position and movement in upper limbs and report your findings.

Domains tested: Cognitive, psychomotor, affective and communication

S. no.	Steps	Marks	R. no. 1	R. no. 2	R. no. 3
A.	**Checklist**				
1.	Takes proper consent to perform the procedure	1			
2.	Orients the patient about the procedure in local language	1			
3.	Gives instruction to the subject to recognize the position at which the limb is moved and to recognize the direction of movement	1			
4.	Asks the subject to close his eyes.	2			
5.	Moves the finger or hand up or down and asks the position at which the finger/ hand is kept.	2			
6.	Makes a particular movement and then places the upper limb at a particular stance and asks the subject to imitate the final stance of the limb	2			
7.	Compares the same sense of position and movement on the opposite limb	1			
8.	Narrates the findings to the observer	1			
B.	**Assessment of Professional Behavior**				
1.	Informs subject regarding completion of procedure and thanks the subject	1			
	Total Marks	**12**			
	Correction Factor				
	Final Score				
	Global Rating: 1. Poor; 2. Unsatisfactory; 3. Satisfactory; 4. Good; 5. Excellent				

Observer's Comment (based on general observation):

Signature of Observer

Response stations:
1. Enumerate various sensations.
2. Enumerate various tactile receptors.
3. Which tract carries sense of position.
4. Draw diagram of tract carrying this sensation.

Central Nervous System: Sensory System   Date:

Station no. 61: Examine the given subject for vibration sense and report your findings.

Domains tested: Cognitive, psychomotor, affective and communication

S. no.	Steps	Marks	R. no. 1	R. no. 2	R. no. 3
A.	**Checklist**				
1.	Takes proper consent to perform the procedure	1			
2.	Orients the patient about the procedure in local language	1			
3.	Selects 128 Hz tuning fork	1			
4.	Instructs subject to raise his hand when he stops feeling the vibration	1			
5.	Asks the subject to close his eyes.	2			
6.	Makes the tuning fork vibrate without touching the blades of the tuning fork	1			
7.	Places the foot of the tuning fork on any bony prominence of the subject	2			
8.	Places the tuning fork on own corresponding bony prominence after the subject stops feeling the sensation	2			
9.	Compares the same sense of vibration on the opposite limb	1			
10.	Narrates the findings to the observer	1			
B.	**Assessment of Professional Behavior**				
1.	Informs subject regarding completion of procedure and thanks the subject	1			
	Total Marks	**14**			
	Correction Factor				
	Final Score				
	Global Rating: 1. Poor; 2. Unsatisfactory; 3. Satisfactory; 4. Good; 5. Excellent				
Observer's Comment (based on general observation):					
Signature of Observer					

Response stations:
1. Enumerate various sensations
2. Enumerate various tactile receptors
3. Which tract carries sensation of vibration
4. Draw diagram of tract carrying this sensation.

Central Nervous System: Sensory System   Date:

Station no. 62: Examine the given subject for sense of superficial pain on forearm anterior aspect and report your findings.

Domains tested: Cognitive, psychomotor, affective and communication

S. no.	Steps	Marks	R. no. 1	R. no. 2	R. no. 3
A.	**Checklist**				
1.	Takes proper consent to perform the procedure	1			
2.	Orients the patient about the procedure in local language	1			
3.	Asks the subject to close his eyes	2			
4.	Lightly pricks the skin of a dermatome of forehead or manubrium sterni and asks whether the subject feels sharpness or pain	2			
5.	Lightly pricks the skin on forearm with the intensity of pain and not sharpness	2			
6.	Compares with the same dermatome on the opposite side of the forearm	2			
7.	Narrates the findings to the observer	1			
B.	**Assessment of Professional Behavior**				
1.	Informs subject regarding completion of procedure and thanks the subject	1			
	Total Marks	**12**			
	Correction Factor				
	Final Score				
	Global Rating: 1. Poor; 2. Unsatisfactory; 3. Satisfactory; 4. Good; 5. Excellent				
Observer's Comment (based on general observation):					
Signature of Observer					

Response stations:
1. Enumerate various sensations.
2. Enumerate various tactile receptors.
3. Which tract carries sensation of pain?
4. Draw diagram of tract carrying this sensation.
5. What is referred pain?

Central Nervous System: Sensory System Date:

Station no. 63: Examine the given subject for sense of deep pain and report your findings.

Domains tested: Cognitive, psychomotor, affective and communication

S. no.	Steps	Marks	R. no. 1	R. no. 2	R. no. 3
A.	**Checklist**				
1.	Takes proper consent to perform the procedure	1			
2.	Orients the patient about the procedure in local language	1			
3.	Asks the subject to close his eyes	2			
4.	Squeezes the Achilles tendon till pain is produced	2			
5.	Repeats the procedure on other limb	1			
6.	Narrates the findings to the observer	1			
B.	**Assessment of Professional Behavior**				
1.	Informs subject regarding completion of procedure and thanks the subject	1			
	Total Marks	**9**			
	Correction Factor				
	Final Score				
	Global Rating: 1. Poor; 2. Unsatisfactory; 3. Satisfactory; 4. Good; 5. Excellent				
Observer's Comment (based on general observation):					
Signature of Observer					

Response stations:
1. Enumerate various sensations.
2. Enumerate various tactile receptors.
3. Which tract carries sensation of pain?
4. Draw diagram of tract carrying this sensation.
5. What is referred pain?
6. What is gate control theory of pain?

Central Nervous System: Sensory System   Date:

Station no. 64: Examine the given subject for sense of stereognosis and report your findings.

Domains tested: Psychomotor, affective and communication

S. no.	Steps	Marks	R. no. 1	R. no. 2	R. no. 3
A.	**Checklist**				
1.	Takes proper consent to perform the procedure	1			
2.	Orients the patient about the procedure in local language	1			
3.	Asks the subject to close his eyes	2			
4.	Asks the subject to identify the familiar object placed in one hand of the subject by palpating it	2			
5.	Repeats the handing over of a familiar object in the opposite hand	1			
6.	Narrates the findings to the observer	1			
B.	**Assessment of Professional Behavior**				
1.	Informs subject regarding completion of procedure and thanks the subject	1			
	Total Marks	**9**			
	Correction Factor				
	Final Score				
	Global Rating: 1. Poor; 2. Unsatisfactory; 3. Satisfactory; 4. Good; 5. Excellent				
	Observer's Comment (based on general observation):				
	Signature of Observer				

Response stations:
1. Enumerate various sensations.
2. Enumerate various tactile receptors.
3. Which tract carries sensation of stereognosis.
4. Draw diagram of tract carrying this sensation.

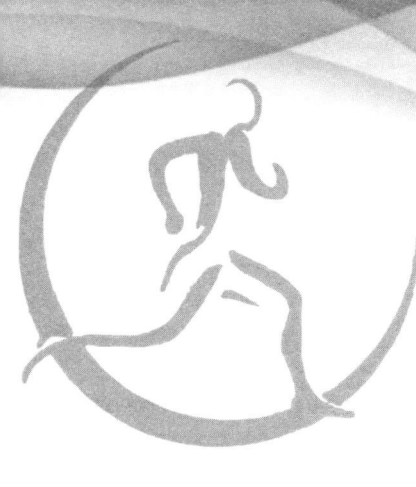

OSPE

OSPE Stations: Hematology

65. An 8-year-old boy was on cytotoxic therapy for malignancy. On his follow-up, he was advised a blood investigation that generally decreases in such condition exposing the child for opportunistic infections
Dilute the blood for performing the investigation (blood sample given)

66. A 16-year-old female, on a pure vegetarian diet, had complaints of tingling numbness, easy fatigability and blackish discoloration of knuckles
Dilute the blood for performing the investigation that would help in diagnosis (blood sample given)

67. A 5-year-old girl had history of passing worms in stool, poor appetite and easy fatigability
Charge the Neubauer's chamber for performing the count related to this condition

68. An adult male presented with high grade fever and chills. He had abscess in right thigh medial aspect
Charge the Neubauer's chamber for performing the blood investigation that will support the diagnosis

69. Perform the blood group investigation of the given sample (red cell suspension provided)

Hematology

Hematology: Date:

Station no. 65: An 8-year-old boy was on cytotoxic therapy for malignancy. On his follow-up, he was advised a blood investigation that generally decreases in such condition exposing the child for opportunistic infections.

Dilute the blood for performing the investigation (blood sample given)

Domains tested: Cognitive, psychomotor

S. no.	Steps	Marks	R. no. 1	R. no. 2	R. no. 3
A.	**Checklist**				
1.	Takes adequate white blood cell (WBC) diluting fluid in a watch glass	1			
2.	Selects WBC pipette	1.5			
3.	Ensures that the WBC pipette is clean and dry	1			
4.	Pipettes blood up to 0.5 mark of pipette	1.5			
5.	Wipes the tip of the pipette	1			
6.	Sucks the diluting fluid up to 101 mark of pipette	2			
7.	Holds the pipette horizontally, gently mixes the contents of the bulb and places the pipette on the table	2			
	Total Marks	**10**			
	Correction Factor				
	Final Score				
	Global Rating: 1. Poor; 2. Unsatisfactory; 3. Satisfactory; 4. Good; 5. Excellent				
Observer's Comment (based on general observation):					
Signature of Observer					

Prerequisites:
- Adequate number of WBC and RBC pipettes, watch glasses should be placed in a tray.
- Turk's fluid, Hayem's/any other RBC diluting fluid used in the lab, Leishman's stain to be kept on the station.
- Artificial blood should be prepared to avoid infection.
- Adequate amount of tissue paper should be placed at the station.

Hematology: Date:

Station no. 66: A 16-year-old female, on a pure vegetarian diet had complaints of tingling numbness, easy fatigability and blackish discoloration of knuckles.

Dilute the blood for performing the investigation that would help in diagnosis (Blood sample given).

Domains tested: Cognitive, psychomotor

S. no.	Steps	Marks	R. no. 1	R. no. 2	R. no. 3
A.	**Checklist**				
1.	Takes adequate red blood cell (RBC) diluting fluid in a watch glass	1			
2.	Selects RBC pipette	1.5			
3.	Ensures that the RBC pipette is clean and dry	1			
4.	Pipettes blood up to 0.5 mark of pipette	1.5			
5.	Wipes the tip of the pipette	1			
6.	Sucks the diluting fluid up to 101 mark of pipette	2			
7.	Holds the pipette horizontally, gently mixes the contents of the bulb and places the pipette on the table	2			
	Total Marks	**10**			
	Correction Factor				
	Final Score				
	Global Rating: 1. Poor; 2. Unsatisfactory; 3. Satisfactory; 4. Good; 5. Excellent				
Observer's Comment (based on general observation):					
Signature of Observer					

Prerequisites:
- Adequate number of WBC and RBC pipettes, watch glasses should be placed in a tray.
- Turk's fluid, Hayem's/any other RBC diluting fluid used in the lab, Leishman's stain to be kept on the station.
- Artificial blood should be prepared to avoid infection.
- Adequate amount of tissue paper should be placed at the station.

Hematology: Date:

Station no. 67: A 5-year-old girl had history of passing worms in stool, poor appetite and easy fatigability.

Charge the Neubauer's chamber for performing the count related to this condition.

Domains tested: Cognitive, psychomotor

S. no.	Steps	Marks	R. no. 1	R. no. 2	R. no. 3
A.	**Checklist**				
1.	Cleans the Neubauer's chamber	0.5			
2.	Cleans the coverslip	0.5			
3.	Places the coverslip on the Neubauer's chamber platform	1			
4.	Mixes the contents of the red blood cell (RBC) pipette bulb thoroughly	1.5			
5.	Discards two drops of fluid from pipette before charging	1.5			
6.	Places the tip of RBC pipette touching the edge of the coverslip	2			
7.	Allows the diluted blood to flow by capillary action under the coverslip.	2			
8.	Takes care that the diluted blood does not overflow the gutters or contain air bubbles.	1			
	Total Marks	**10**			
	Correction Factor				
	Final Score				
	Global Rating: 1. Poor; 2. Unsatisfactory; 3. Satisfactory; 4. Good; 5. Excellent				
Observer's Comment (based on general observation):					
Signature of Observer					

Prerequisites:
- Adequate number of filled WBC and RBC pipettes should be placed in a tray.
- Adequate number of Neubauer's chambers and coverslips to be kept on the station.
- Adequate amount of tissue paper should be placed at the station.

Hematology: Date:

Station no. 68: An adult male presented with high grade fever and chills. He had abscess in right thigh medial aspect.

Charge the Neubauer's chamber for performing the blood investigation that will support the diagnosis.

Domains tested: Cognitive, psychomotor

S. no.	Steps	Marks	R. no. 1	R. no. 2	R. no. 3
A.	**Checklist**				
1.	Cleans the Neubauer's chamber	0.5			
2.	Cleans the coverslip	0.5			
3.	Places the coverslip on the Neubauer's chamber platform	1			
4.	Mixes the contents of the white blood cell (WBC) pipette bulb thoroughly	1.5			
5.	Discards two drops of fluid from pipette before charging	1.5			
6.	Places the tip of WBC pipette touching the edge of the coverslip	2			
7.	Allows the diluted blood to flow by capillary action under the coverslip	2			
8.	Takes care that the diluted blood does not overflow the gutters or contain air bubbles	1			
	Total Marks	**10**			
	Correction Factor				
	Final Score				
	Global Rating: 1. Poor; 2. Unsatisfactory; 3. Satisfactory; 4. Good; 5. Excellent				
Observer's Comment (based on general observation):					
Signature of Observer					

Prerequisites:
- Adequate number of filled WBC and RBC pipettes should be placed in a tray.
- Adequate number of Neubauer's chambers and coverslips to be kept on the station.
- Adequate amount of tissue paper should be placed at the station.

Hematology: Date:

Station no. 69: Perform the blood group investigation of the given sample (red cell suspension provided).

Domains tested: Psychomotor

S. no.	Steps	Marks	R. no. 1	R. no. 2	R. no. 3
A.	**Checklist**				
1.	Selects two slides marked A, B and C, D	1			
2.	Places a drop of red cell suspension on A, B, C and D	1			
3.	Adds a drop of anti-A serum on 'A'	1.5			
4.	Adds a drop of anti-B serum on 'B'	1.5			
5.	Adds a drop of anti-D serum on 'D'	1.5			
6.	Adds a drop of 0.9% normal saline on 'C'	1.5			
7.	Mixes the red cell suspension with the anti-sera using separate edges of glass slide/ by gently shaking the slides	1			
8.	Narrates the findings to the observer	1			
	Total Marks	**10**			
	Correction Factor				
	Final Score				
	Global Rating: 1. Poor; 2. Unsatisfactory; 3. Satisfactory; 4. Good; 5. Excellent				
Observer's Comment (based on general observation):					
Signature of Observer					

Prerequisites:
- Adequate quantity of anti-sera, 0.9% normal saline solution should be placed in a tray.
- Adequate amount of red cell suspension to be kept on the station.
- Adequate number of marked slides, plain slides to be kept on the station.
- Adequate amount of tissue paper should be placed at the station.

Photographs

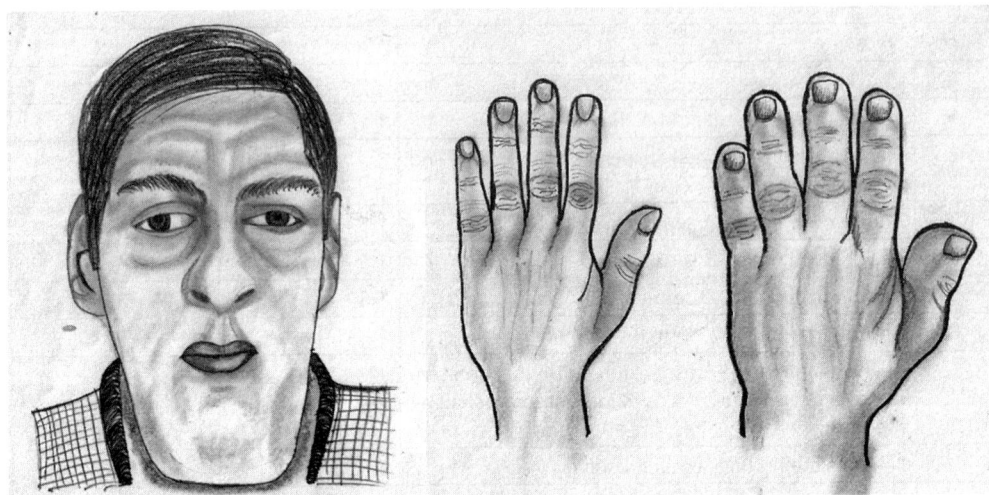

Figure 1

1. Identify the condition.
2. Give the cause for this condition.
3. Enumerate any two features of this condition.
4. Write the location of lesion in visual pathway and the resulting feature in eye.

Key: Acromegaly

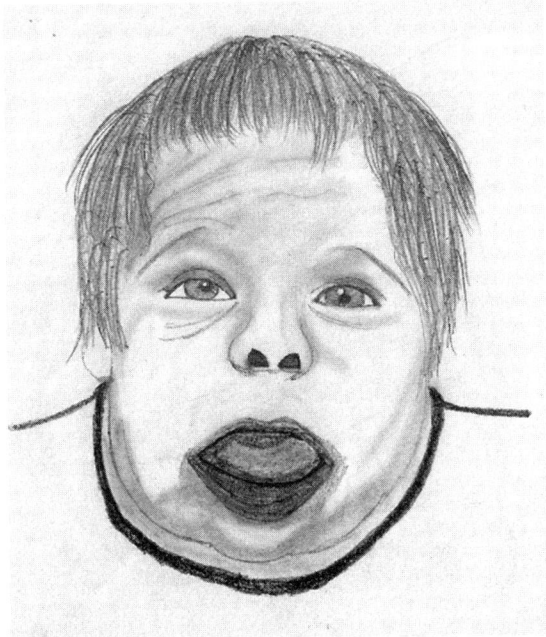

Figure 2

1. Identify the condition.
2. Give the cause for this condition.
3. Enumerate any two features of this condition.
4. Write the effect on mental growth of the baby.

Key: Cretinism

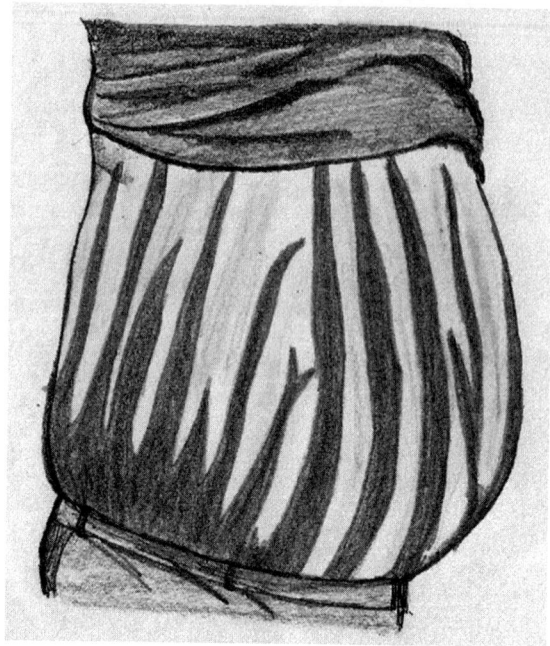

Figure 3

1. Identify the condition.
2. Give the cause for this condition.
3. Enumerate any two features of this condition.
4. Describe the cause of diabetes in this condition.

Key: Cushing's syndrome

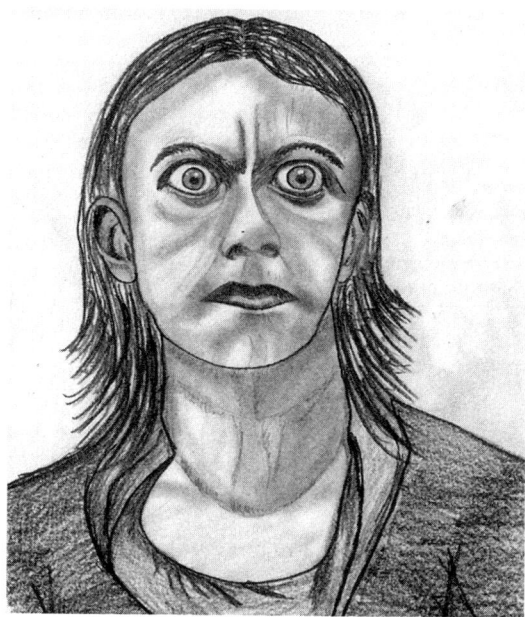

Figure 4

1. Identify the condition.
2. Give the cause for this condition.
3. Enumerate any two features of this condition.
4. Describe the cause for the eye features.

Key: Hyperthyroidism

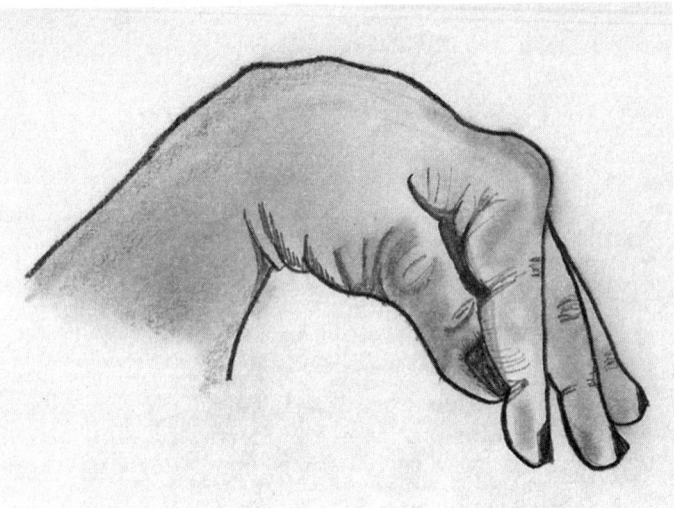

Figure 5

1. Identify the condition.
2. Give the cause for this condition.
3. Enumerate any two features of this condition.
4. Upon tapping the facial nerve in front of the tragus, there is twitching on that side of the face. Identify the sign.

Key: Carpal spasm

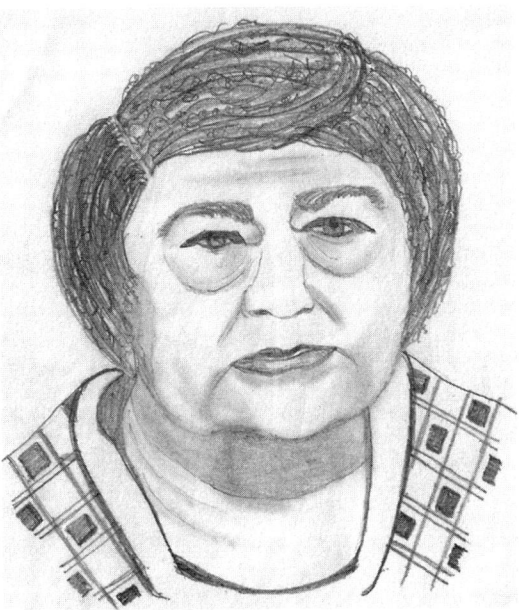

Figure 6

1. Identify the condition.
2. Give the cause for this condition.
3. Enumerate any two features of this condition.
4. Describe the gastrointestinal system changes in this condition.

Key: Myxedema

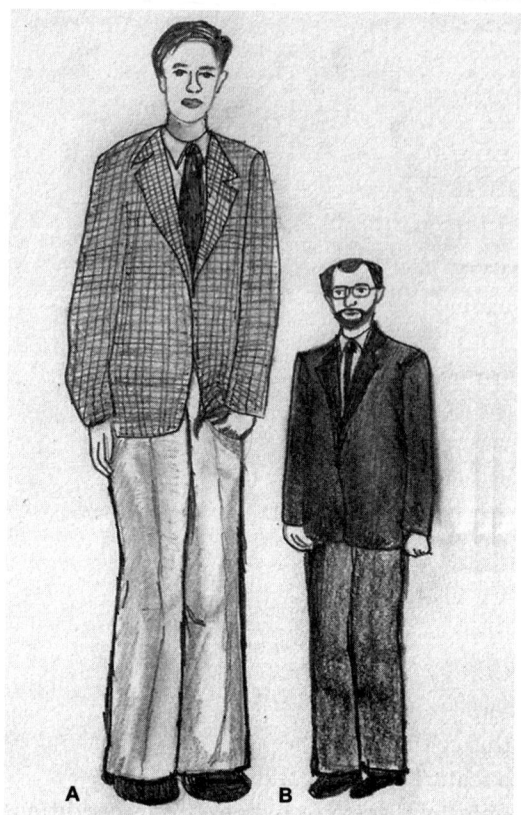

Figure 7

1. Identify A the condition
2. Give the cause for this condition
3. Enumerate any two features of this condition

Key: Gigantism

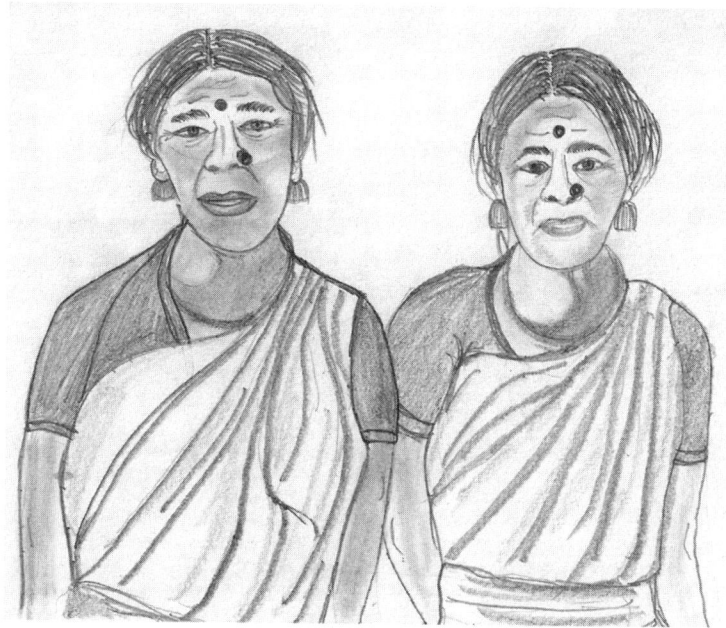

Figure 8

1. Identify the condition.
2. Give the cause for this condition.
3. Enumerate any two features of this condition.
4. Enumerate the steps of synthesis of the hormone causing this condition.

Key: Endemic goiter

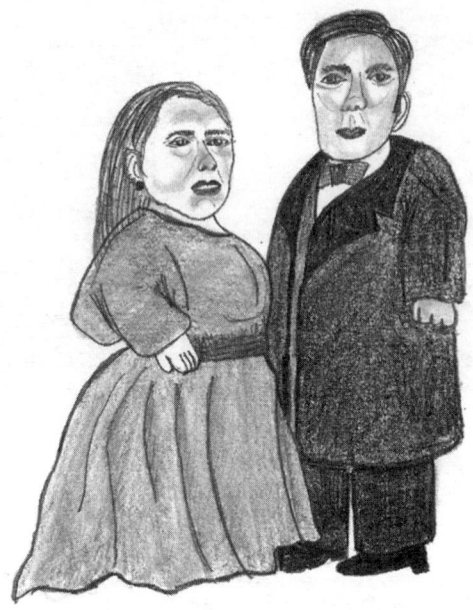

Figure 9

1. Identify the condition.
2. Give the cause for this condition.
3. Enumerate any two features of this condition.

Key: Dwarfism

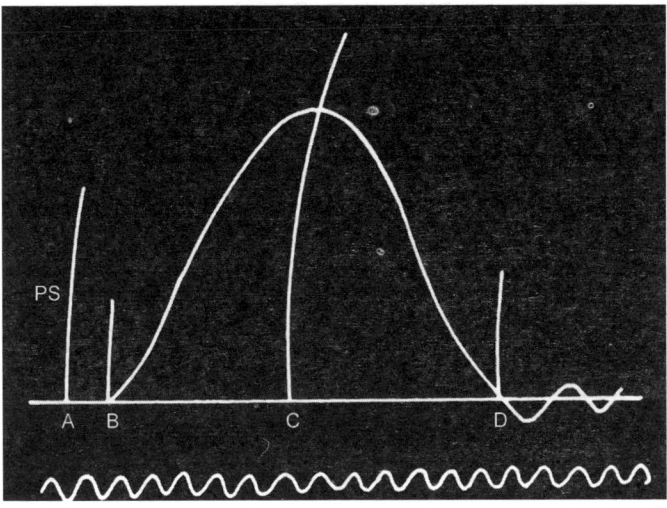

Figure 10

1. Identify the graph and comment.
2. What is the importance of this graph?
3. Name the periods from A – B, B–C and C–D and write their causes.
4. Enumerate the causes of latent phase.

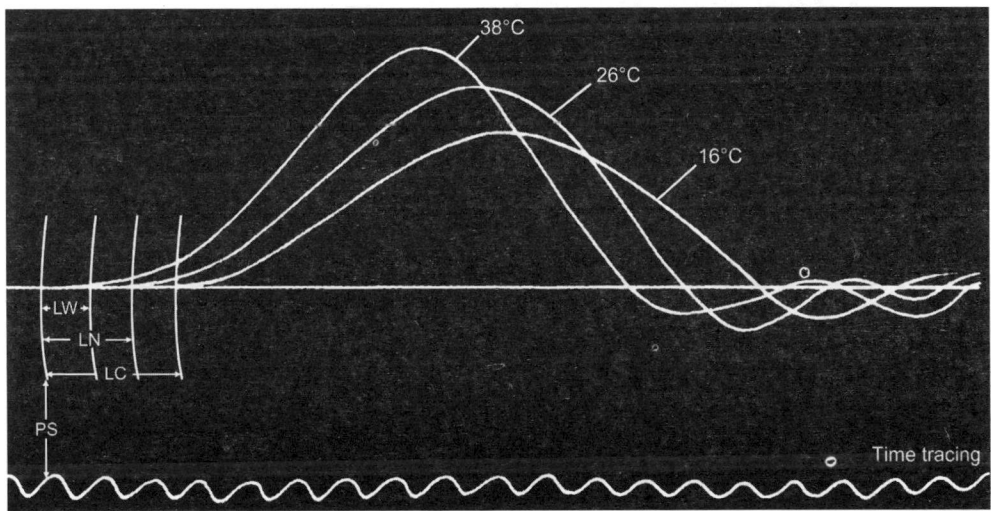

Figure 11

1. Identify the graph.
2. What is the effect of temperature?
3. What is heat and cold rigor?

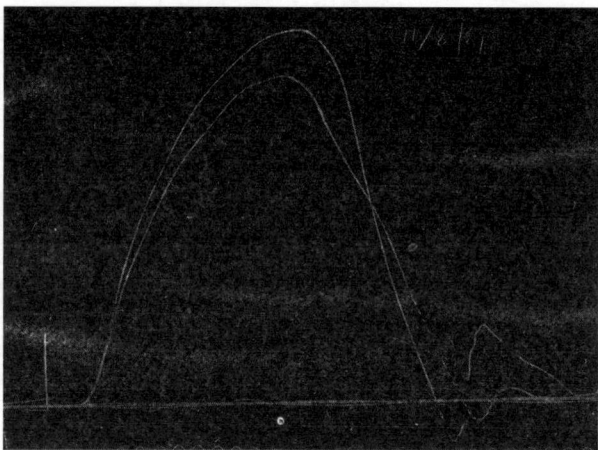

Figure 12

1. Identify the graph.
2. What is Starling's law?
3. Give one example of these conditions in the heart.
4. What is SEC and PEC?

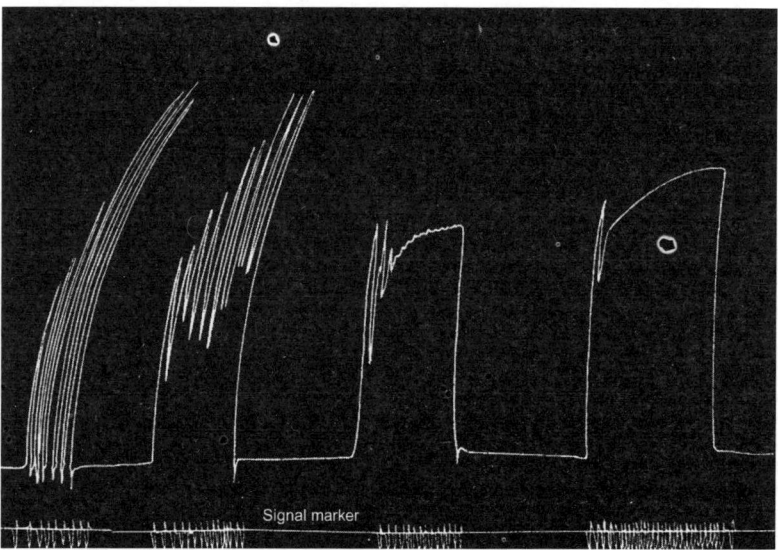

Figure 13

1. Identify the graph.
2. What is clonus?
3. Differentiate between tetanus, treppe, incomplete tetanus.
4. What is the stimulus frequency to tetanize the muscle?

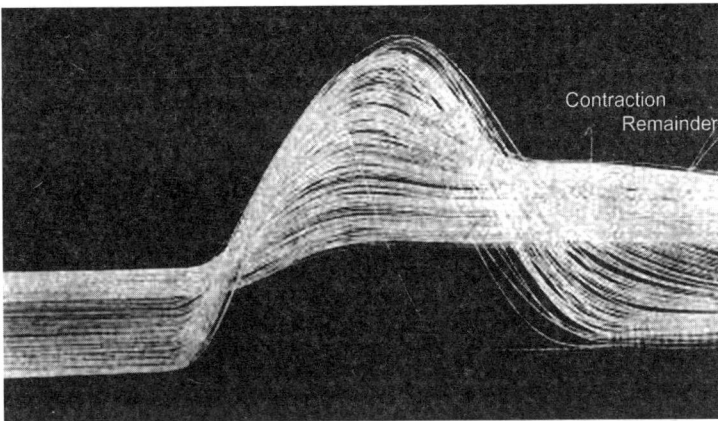

Figure 14

1. Identify the graph. What is contraction remainder?
2. What are the various causes of given phenomenon?
3. What are the causes of this phenomenon/property in pithed and non-pithed animal?

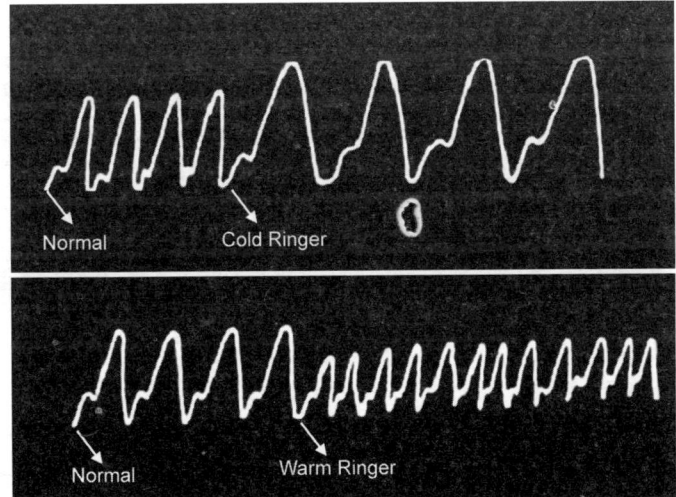

Figure 15

1. Identify the graph.
2. What is the effect of hot and cold Ringer solution on SA node?

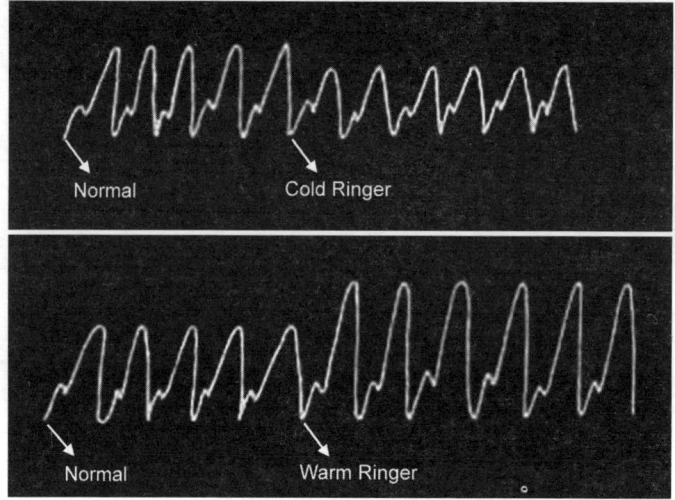

Figure 16

1. Identify the graph.
2. What is the effect of hot and cold Ringer solution on ventricles?

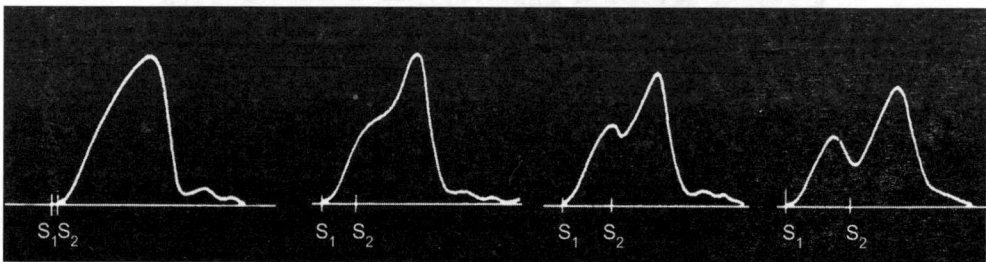

Figure 17

1. Identify the graph.
2. What is refractory period?
3. What is quantal summation?

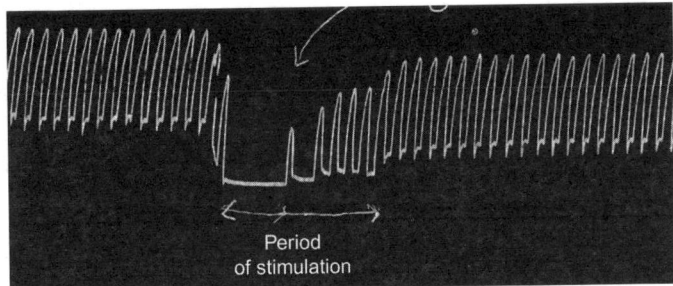

Figure 18

1. Identify the graph and comment.
2. What is the mechanism of cardiac inhibition?
3. What are the causes of escape in pithed and non-pithed animal?

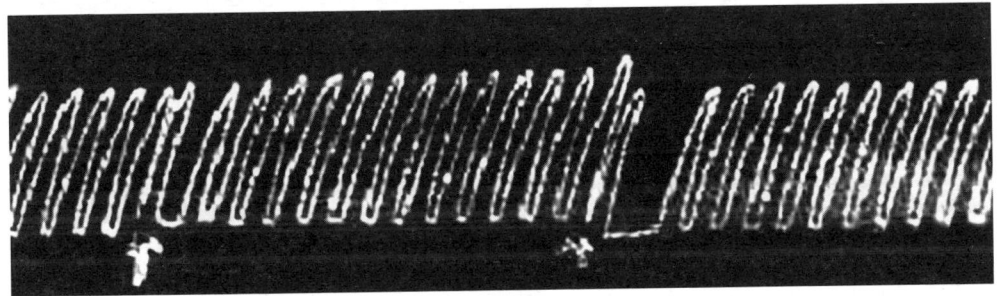

Figure 19

1. Identify graph.
2. Which property of cardiac muscle is demonstrated by this graph?
3. What is the cause of extra-systole in normal life?
4. What is the cause of pause in the given graph?

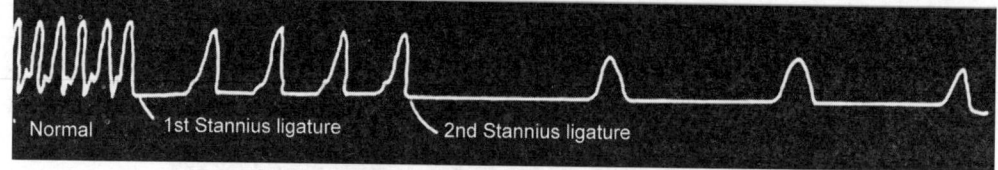

Figure 20

1. Which property of cardiac muscle is demonstrated by this graph?
2. Can we apply Stannius ligature in human heart? Why?
3. What is the cause of idioventricular rhythm?

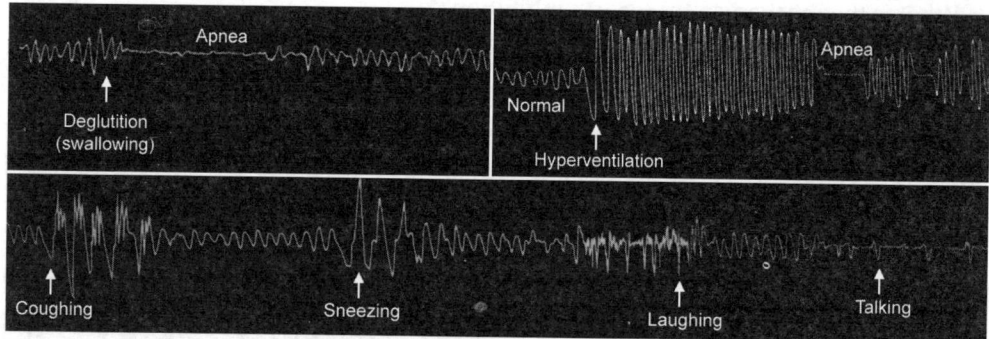

Figure 21

1. Identify the graph and what are the effects of various activities?
2. What is the cause of deglutition apnea?
3. What is the cause of hyperventilation apnea?

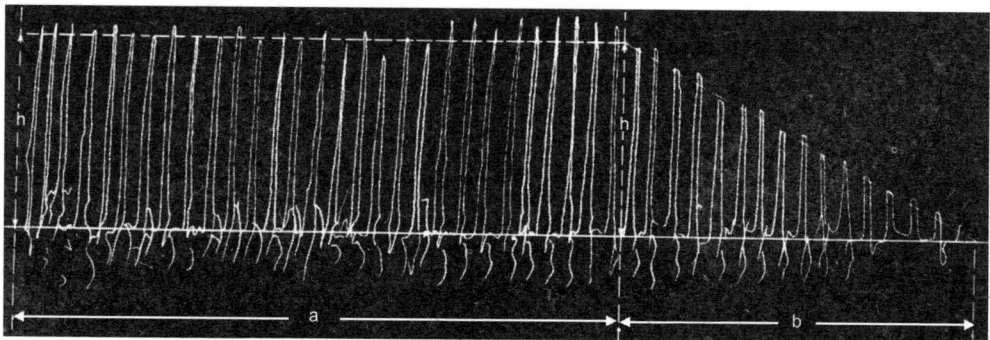

Figure 22

1. Identify the graph.
2. Calculate work done from given graph. (Weight = 2 kg)
3. Whether the given phenomenon is reversible or irreversible?
4. What are the various sites of fatigue?

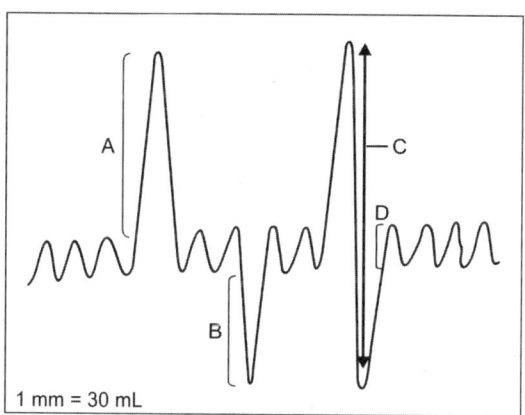

Figure 23

1. Identify the graph. What is A, B, C, and D?
2. Define and calculate the tidal volume and vital capacity.
3. Which lung volume and capacity cannot be calculated by this graph?

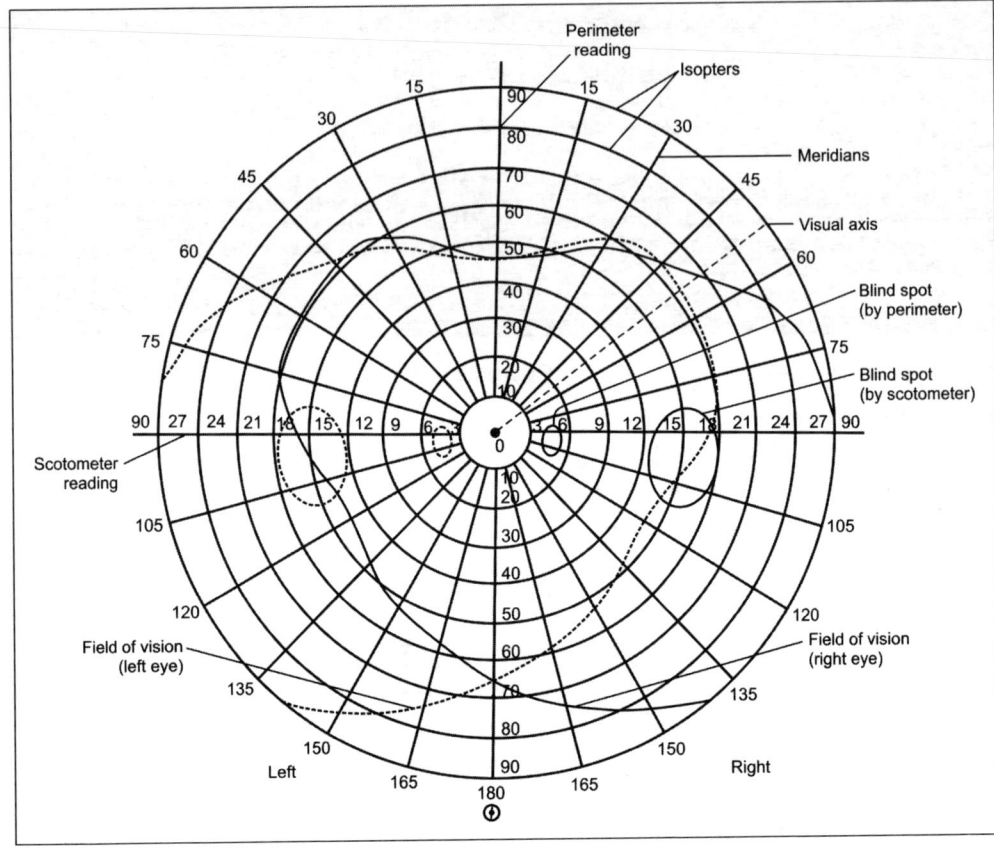

Figure 24

1. Identify the graph.
2. What is physiological blind spot? What is its location?
3. Give the normal field of vision in all the quadrants.
4. What are the factors affecting field of vision?
5. Trace the visual pathway and name the field defects.
6. What is the field of vision for red color?

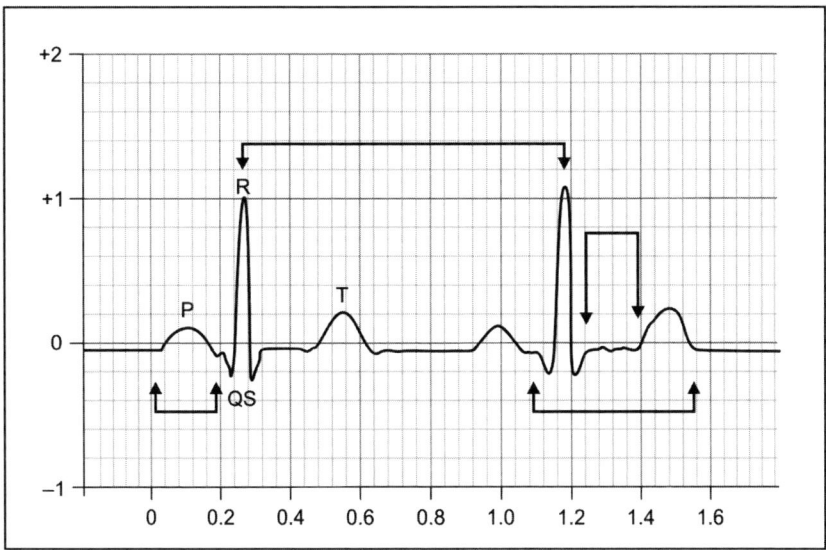

Figure 25

1. Write down the causes of various waves.
2. Calculate PR interval. What is its significance?
3. Calculate the heart rate.
4. Calculate the amplitude and duration of P wave.
5. What is the significance of ST segment?
6. What is the duration of QRS complex?

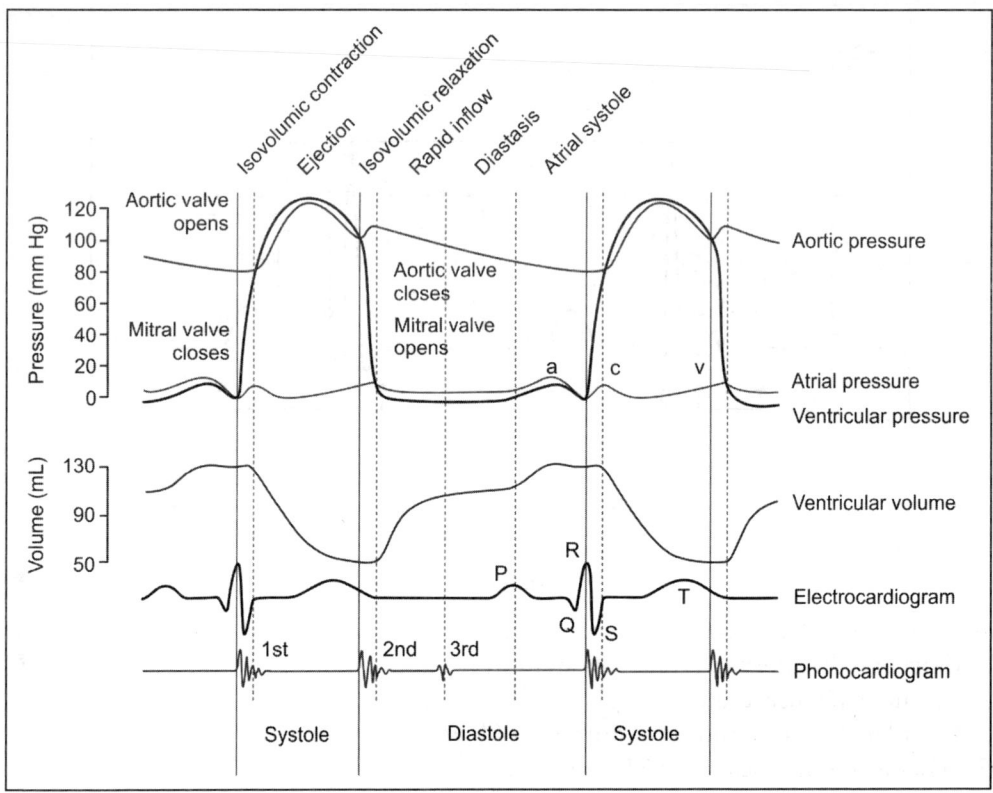

Figure 26

1. Identify the graph.
2. During which phase of cardiac cycle, there is maximum rise in pressure in left ventricle.
3. How much is end diastolic volume in ventricles?

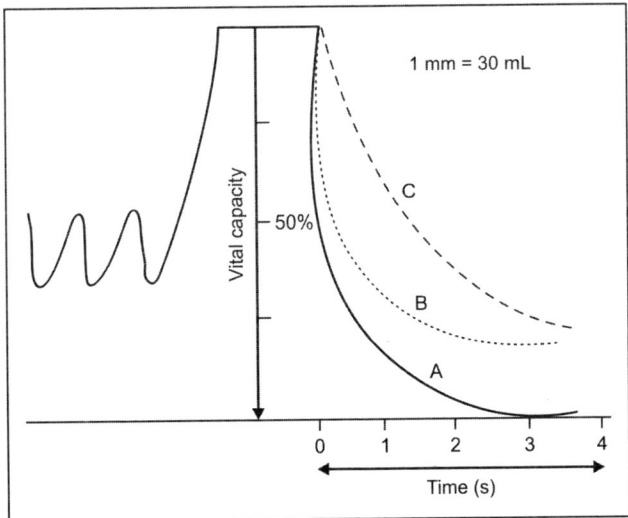

Figure 27

1. Identify the graph. What is timed vital capacity?
2. Calculate FEV_1. What is its significance?
3. Name the conditions in which it decreases.
4. Label the curves A, B, and C.

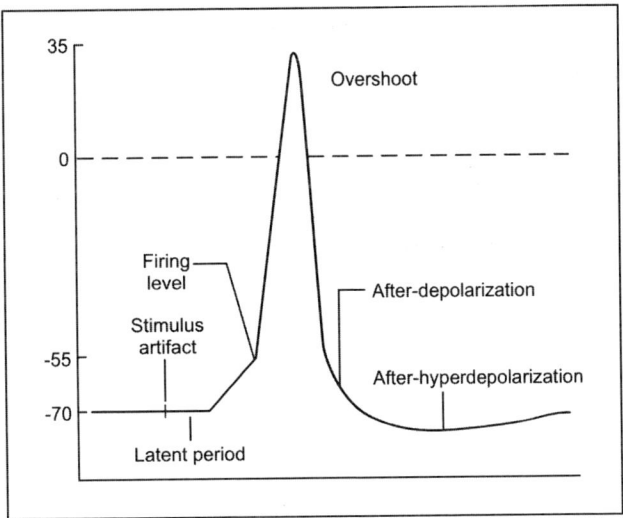

Figure 28

1. Identify the graph.
2. What is the cause of stimulus artifact?
3. What is the cause of depolarization?
4. What is the cause of latent period?
5. What is the cause of repolarization?

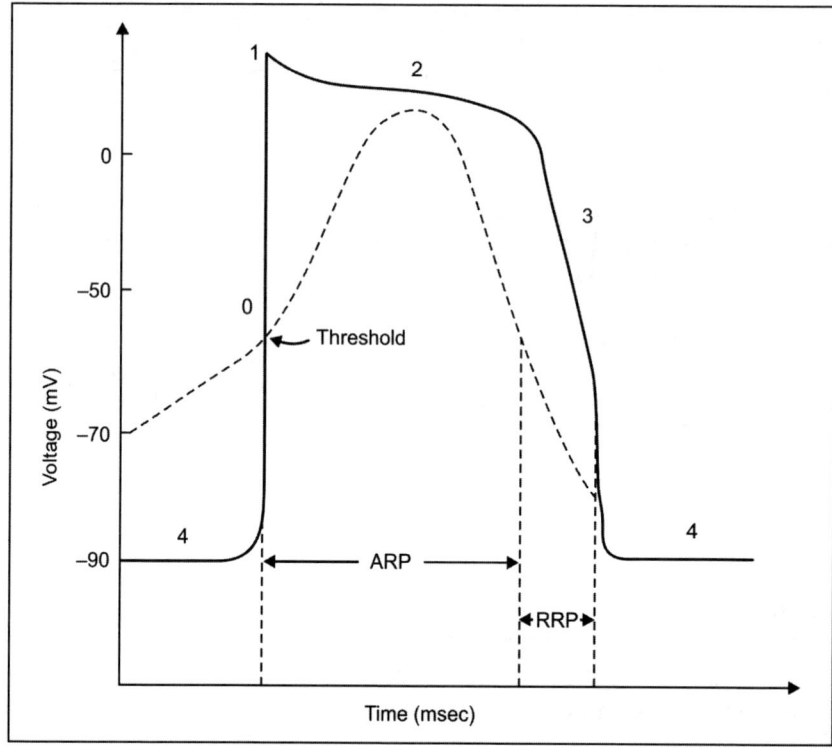

Figure 29

1. Identify the graph.
2. Label the different phases from 0–4.
3. What is the ionic basis of phase 2.
4. Name the dotted and solid curves.
5. What is ARP and RRP?
6. What is the ionic basis of phase 0.

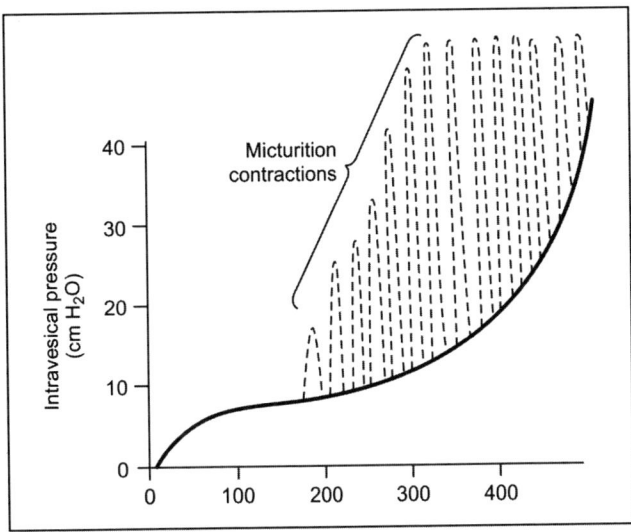

Figure 30

1. Identify the graph and comment.
2. What is the minimum volume for initial urge for micturition?
3. What property of smooth muscle play role in this reflex?

Problem-Solving Questions

Q1. Calculate T_mG from the following data

$[T_mG$ (mg/min)= Filtered load – Excretion rate]
   i. Plasma glucose concentration = 300 mg/100 mL
   ii. GFR = 100 mL/min
   iii. Glucose concentration in urine = 10 mg/mL
   iv. Rate of urine formation = 1 mL/min

Solution:

Formula = T_mG = Filtered rate – Excretion rate
$$(PG \times GFR) - (UG \times V)$$
Solution: T_mG = $(3 \times 100) - (10 \times 1)$
$$= 300 - 10 = 290 \text{ mg/min}$$

Q.2. (a) What is plasma clearance? Name the plasma clearance tests.
(b) Calculate the PAH clearance from the given data. What is its significance?
   i. PAH concentration in plasma = 0.02 mg/mL
   ii. PAH concentration in urine = 14 mg/mL
   iii. Rate of urine formation = 0.9 mL/min

Solution:

Formula: $\dfrac{U \times V}{P} = \dfrac{14 \times 0.9}{0.02} = 630 \text{ mL/min}$

Q. 3. (a) What is plasma clearance? Name the plasma clearance tests.
(b) Calculate the urea clearance from the given data
   i. Urea concentration in plasma = 20 mg/100 mL
   ii. Urea concentration in urine = 10 mg/mL
   iii. Rate of urine formation = 1.2 mL/min

Solution:

Formula: $\dfrac{U \times V}{P} = \dfrac{10 \times 1.2}{0.2 \text{ mg/ml}} = 60 \text{ mL/min}$

Q4. (a) Calculate the net effective filtration pressure from the following data
   i. Hydrostatic pressure in the glomerulus = 60 mm Hg
   ii. Hydrostatic pressure in the Bowman's capsule = 15 mm Hg
   iii. Osmotic pressure in the glomerulus = 30 mm Hg
   iv. Osmotic pressure of the glomerular filtrate = 00 mm Hg

(b) What is autoregulation of RBF and GFR?
Solution:

Net filtration pressure (NFP) = $P_G - P_B - \pi_G$
$$= 60 - 15 - 30 - 0 = 15 \text{ mm Hg}$$

Q5. (a) What is plasma clearance? Name the plasma clearance tests.
(b) Enumerate the substances that are used to measure the GFR and which criteria they should fulfill.

(c) Calculate inulin clearance using following data
    i. Inulin concentration in plasma = 35 mg/100 mL
   ii. Inulin concentration in urine = 25 mg/mL
  iii. Rate of urine formation = 1.4 mL/min
Solution:

Formula: $\dfrac{U \times V}{P} = \dfrac{25 \times 1.4}{0.35 \text{ mg/ml}} = 100 \text{ mL/min}$

Q6. (a) Calculate the dyspneic index from the following data and write your interpretation.
    i. Respiratory rate – 15 /min
   ii. Tidal volume = 500 mL
  iii. MVV = 150 Litre

(b) What is the index at which subject becomes dyspneic at rest?
Solution:

Formula: $\dfrac{MVV - PV}{MVV} \times 100$ where PV = TV × RR

Solution: PV = 500 mL × 15/min = 7500 mL/min = 7.5 L/min

Formula: $\dfrac{MVV - PV}{MVV} \times 100 = \dfrac{150 - 7.5}{150} \times 100 = 95\%$

Q7. (a) Calculate RV and FRC from the given data.
    i. IRV = 3 L
   ii. ERV = 1.8 L
  iii. TV = 0.5 L
  iv. TLC = 6 L

(b) What is the significance of FRC and RV?
Solution:
$$VC = IRV + TV + ERV$$
$$VC = 3 + 0.5 + 1.8 = 5.3$$
$$TLC = VC + RV$$
$$6 = 5.3 + RV$$
$$RV = 6 - 5.3 = 0.7 \text{ L}$$
$$FRC = RV + ERV$$
$$= 0.7 + 1.8 = 2.5 \text{ L}$$

Q8. A subject inhales 1 liter of air and holds his breath with glottis open. At the beginning of inspiration, his esophageal pressure was — 5 cm H_2O and during breath holding it was — 7.5 cm H_2O.
(a) What is the compliance of the lung in this subject?
(b) State one disease in which lung compliance decreases.

Q9. (a) Calculate the lung compliance from the data given below.
    Change in lung volume = 1 L
          Pressure change = 5 cm H_2O
(b) State the conditions in which lungs are more compliant.

Solution:

Formula: $\dfrac{\Delta V}{\Delta P}$

Solution: $\dfrac{1L}{5 \text{ cm of } H_2O} = 0.2 \text{ L/cm of } H_2O$

Q10. (a) What is cardiac output?

(b) Calculate the cardiac output by Fick's principle from the given data.

   i. O_2 concentration in the pulmonary artery is 14 mL/dL.

   ii. O_2 concentration in the brachial artery is 19 mL/dL.

   iii. Oxygen consumption per minute is 250 mL

Solution:

Formula: $\dfrac{250}{0.19 - 0.14} = 250/0.05 = 5000 \text{ mL/min}$

Q11. (a) Calculate the partial pressure of O_2 in the alveoli.

   i. Concentration of O_2 in the alveoli is 15%.

   ii. Water vapor pressure is 47 mm Hg.

b. What is the partial pressure of O_2 in the arterial blood?

Solution:

$$\text{Partial pressure} = \frac{15}{100} \times 760\text{--}47 = 106.75 \text{ mm Hg}$$

Q12. (a) Calculate the partial pressure of O_2 in the ambient air at standard temperature, if the concentration of O_2 in the air is 20%.

(b) What is the partial pressure of O_2 in the arterial blood?

Solution:

$$\text{Partial pressure} = \frac{20}{100} \times 760 = 152 \text{ mm Hg}$$

Q13. (a) What are the methods of measurement of cardiac output?

(b) Calculate the cardiac output by Fick's principle from the given data.

   i. O_2 concentration in the pulmonary artery is 14 mL/dL.

   ii. O_2 concentration in the brachial artery is 19 mL/dL.

   iii. Oxygen consumption per minute is 240 mL

Solution:

Formula: $\dfrac{240}{0.19 - 0.14} = \dfrac{240}{0.05} = 4800 \text{ mL/min}$

Q14. Calculate the dyspneic index of a subject from the following data.

   i. Resting pulmonary ventilation = 6 L/min

   ii. Maximum voluntary ventilation = 100 L/min

Solution:

Formula: $\dfrac{MVV - PV}{MVV} \times 100$

Solution: $\dfrac{100 - 6}{100} \times 100 = 94\%$

Q15. Find out the cardiac output, stroke volume, and cardiac index from the following data.

$$\text{Arterial } O_2 \text{ content} = 19 \text{ mL}/100 \text{ mL}$$
$$\text{Venous } O_2 \text{ content} = 14 \text{ mL}/100 \text{ mL}$$
$$O_2 \text{ consumption} = 270 \text{ mL}/\text{min}$$
$$\text{Surface area} = 1.5 \text{ sq meter}$$
$$\text{Heart rate} = 70 \text{ beats}/\text{min}$$

Solution:

Formula: $\dfrac{270}{0.19-0.14} = \dfrac{270}{0.05} = 5400 \text{ mL}/\text{min}$

Stroke volume: $\dfrac{\text{Cardiac output}}{\text{Heart rate}} = \dfrac{5400}{70} = 77 \text{ mL}$

Cardiac index: $\dfrac{\text{Cardiac output}}{\text{Body surface area}} = \dfrac{5.4}{1.5} = 3.6 \text{ L}/\text{mL}$

Q16. Find out the dead space volume from the following data
  i. Tidal volume = 500 mL
 ii. Alveolar PCO_2 = 40 mm Hg
iii. Expired air PCO_2 = 28 mm Hg

Solution:

$$\text{Dead space} = \text{Tidal volume} \times \dfrac{PCO_2 - PCO_2 \text{ in expired air}}{PCO_2}$$

$$= 500 \times \dfrac{40-28}{40} = 150 \text{ mL}$$

Bibliography

1. Core competencies examined during various skills of Mini CEX; www.abim.org accessed on 1.9.2015 http://www.mmc.nhs.uk/pages/assessment/minicex.

2. Gleeson F. Assessment of Clinical Competence using the Objective Structured Long Examination Record (OSLER), AMEE Medical Education Guide No. 9. Med Teach 1997 19:7–14.

3. Gupta P, Dewan P Singh T. Objective Structured Clinical Examination (OSCE) Revisited. Ind Ped 2010;47: 911-20.

4. Khan KZ, Ramchandran S, Gaunt K, Pushkar P.The Objective Structured Clinical Examination (OSCE): AMEE Guide No. 81. Part I: An historical and theoretical perspective. Med Teach 2013; 35: e1437–e1446.

5. Links for OSCE:
   http://www.oscehome.com/
   http://www.osceskills.com/
   http://en.wikiversity.org/wiki/Category:OSCE

6. Mcmanus IC, Thompson M, Mollon J. Assessment of examiner leniency and stringency ('hawk-dove effect') in the MRCP(UK) clinical examination (PACES) using multi-facet Rasch modelling. BMC Medical Education 2006; 6:42.

7. Miller GE. The assessment of clinical skills/competence/performance. Acad Med. 1990;65:563-7.

8. PMETB Assessment Committee. Developing and Maintaining an Assessment System - a PMETB guide to good practice. Postgraduate Medical Education and Training Board. London; 2007. Available from: http:// www.gmc uk.org/Assessment_good_practice_v0207. pdf_31385949. pdf. Accessed 17 June, 2014.

9. Ponnamperuma GG, Karunathilake IM, Mcaleer S, Davis MH. The long case and its modifications: A literature review. Med Educ 2009;43: 936–941.

10. Rethans J, Norcini J, Baron-Maldonado M, Blackmore D,Jolly B, La Duca T. The relationship between competence and performance: implications for assessing practice performance. Med Educ. 2002; 36:901–9.

11. Smith LJ, Price DA, Houston IB. 1984. Objective structured clinical examination compared with other forms of student assessment. Arch Dis Child 1984;59: 1173–1176.

12. Sood R. Long Case Examination - Can it be Improved. Indian Acad Clin Med 2001;2: 251–255.

13. Tejinder Singh, Anshu. Principles of Assessment in Medical Education: Assessing Professional Competence.

14. Tim Swanwick and NavChana. Workplace assessment for licensing in general practice; British Journal of General Practice, June 2005, 461-467.

15. Walsh K. OSCE. BMJ Learning; 2006 Available from group.bmj.com/products/learning/medical-presentations-2/OSCEs.ppt.

16. Wass V, Van Der Vleuten C. The long case. Med Educ 2004;38: 1176–1180.